D

A Journey Through Medicine

Robert A. Green, M.D.

A DOCTOR'S LESSONS FROM HIS PATIENTS
REFLECTING MEDICAL PRACTICE
DURING THE MID AND LATE TWENTIETH CENTURY

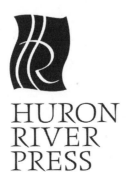

HURON
RIVER
PRESS

10 9 8 7 6 5 4 3 2

ISBN: 978-1-932399-22-6

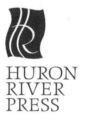

Huron River Press
308½ South State Street
Suite 30
HURON RIVER PRESS
Ann Arbor, MI 48104
www.huronriverpress.com

Printed in the United States of America.

LIBRARY OF CONGRESS CATALOGING-IN-PUBLICATION DATA

Green, Robert A., 1925-
A journey through medicine : a doctor's lessons from his patients reflecting medical practice during the mid and late twentieth century / by Robert A. Green.
  p. ; cm.
  ISBN 1-932399-22-4
  1. Green, Robert A., 1925- 2. Internists--United States--Biography.
I. Title.
  [DNLM: 1. Green, Robert A., 1925- 2. Physicians--United States--Personal Narratives. 3. History, 20th Century--United States--Personal Narratives.
WZ 100 G797j 2009]
  R153.G74 2009
  610.92--dc22
  [B]   2009001065

To my patients, who were major contributors to my education.

To my late wife Lila, with whom I shared the adventure of life.

And to the memory of Dr. Frederic B. Loomis,
in whose footsteps I follow.

Acknowledgements

- to my colleagues, for their support

- to my students, residents and fellows, whose questions, opinions and challenges were seminal in the development of my teaching principles

- to the Ann Arbor Observer, where a few of these vignettes were published in slightly different form

- to Dana Benningfield, my editor, for her remarkably creative help

- and to Steve and Shira Klein, my publishers at Huron River Press

Table of Contents

Preface

Doctors often talk among themselves about their "great cases." They usually are referring to instances of rarity, or unusual findings, or unexpected developments: purely medical aspects of a patient's illness. Although the reader will find some of these among my vignettes, other stories emphasize the fact that my interest has more often centered around the human being involved in the illness and the relationship that consequently developed. And it is the lessons learned from these relationships that have made certain encounters worthy of retelling.

A colleague who reviewed portions of this manuscript observed that it contains many stories revealing errors of judgment in diagnosis and treatment, rather than successes. He said it almost appears that I was wrong more often than right. His observation is correct, not because such outcomes were more common in my practice than the successes, but because my mistakes always allowed greater opportunity for learning. In medicine, when a patient responds exactly as expected, principles are confirmed, but one learns nothing new. When something goes wrong or differently than expected, valuable lessons are imprinted in one's mind and, hopefully, applied to future scenarios. And so it should not be surprising that in this memoir of lessons learned, my errors are (or were) frequent. Please accept that the mistakes described herein are the exception, rather than the norm, during my fifty-seven years of practicing medicine.

The names of the patients have been changed, but all the incidents are presented exactly as they happened.

Introduction

I started college in the fall of 1942 at Harvard. America had recently entered World War II. I enlisted in the Naval Reserve, thinking it my best chance to be able to complete my undergraduate, and perhaps even my medical education, without being drafted. After a year the Navy called me and others like me to active duty. It was, thus, in uniform that I completed my next two terms in February 1944, as Harvard was then on a war-time accelerated schedule. At that point our group of Naval pre-meds was assembled. Some pre-meds were to be sent to medical school immediately. Others were to wait until opportunities became available. Still others were told that medical school was unlikely and were given the choice of attending dental school, or midshipmen's school to become naval line officers, or of becoming pharmacist's mates—hospital corpsmen or "medics"—in the regular Navy. I was in this third group and chose to become a pharmacist's mate. There still existed a small possibility that I might be sent on to medical school if positions opened up or if naval needs changed, but I knew it was a long shot. The possibility of death in action seemed more likely than medical school, and the possibility of becoming a physician, an unlikely dream.

I was obviously depressed. In an attempt to cheer me up, my roommate, Larry Creshkoff, reminded me of an article we had read in *Reader's Digest*. It told the story of a young man named Frederic Loomis who had had his medical education interrupted by family financial pressures, forcing him to spend years—a decade, in fact—

mining in Alaska during the Klondike gold rush. Then one day Loomis encountered some Ivy League professors who convinced him to resume his education. He did. Loomis eventually became a famous obstetrician/ gynecologist and noted author. If he could do it, Larry suggested, surely I could too. A great story; it did little to change my mood.

Six months later I was a corpsman at the Naval Hospital in Oakland, California. One beautiful Sunday morning I was on the road hitchhiking, open to going wherever chance might take me. I was picked up by a woman, her daughter, and her elderly husband. Conversation ensued, and after a while I realized the elderly gentleman was none other than Dr. Loomis himself! I ended up spending that day with him and his extended family in Palo Alto. That marked the beginning of a friendship, and I enjoyed the family's gracious hospitality many times after that at their lovely home in the Piedmont district of Oakland. It was then that I became familiar with Dr. Loomis's charming books: *Consultation Room* and *The Bond Between Us*. I later realized he was responsible for helping to popularize the poignant phrase "Enjoy yourself; it is later than you think," which appeared in his piece, "In a Chinese Garden."

Nineteen forty-four ended with Navy orders for me to attend medical school at the University of Illinois. Much later, on the faculty at the University of Michigan Medical School, I was thrilled to realize that it was Michigan from which Dr. Loomis had left for Alaska, and Michigan to which he had returned not only for medical school but for his specialty training. Recently, one of Dr. Loomis's grandchildren, Lee Sims, published a volume about his grandfather entitled, *Doctor Preacher Author Teacher*. It depicts Loomis as the positive force he was in many people's lives. I, for one, am forever grateful for our chance encounter—a memory that will remain with me forever—and for the significant influence he has exerted on my own life and medical career ever since.

Pharmacist's Mate

M y "medical career" begins with my early departure from college in February 1944. Along with other premed students, I was sent as an apprentice seaman for basic training to Sampson, New York, more aptly referred to as "boot camp." Shortly before our training ended we received our new military rankings. The lowest corpsman ranking was Hospital Apprentice Second Class, followed by First Class. Moving on up the ladder, one became a Pharmacist's mate, third class ("PhM 3c"). Despite the fact that we were untrained, we were designated as PhM 3c's. Normally, one would be proud to receive a higher ranking, but we found ourselves sobered and concerned. We all knew a lot of organic chemistry and a good deal of biology, but our practical knowledge of caring for the sick or wounded was basically nonexistent. What would be expected of us in the field? To say we were anxious would be an understatement. ·

After we completed boot camp, our expectation that we would be assigned to hospitals on the East coast proved unfounded; instead, our troop train moved inexorably west, though we were not told where we were going. To our great relief, rather than being immediately shipped overseas, many of us were assigned to the naval hospital in Oakland, California, colloquially known as "Oak Knoll."

The morning after we arrived, we were taken to Staff Personnel to be given our initial assignments. I stepped up to a desk behind which sat

1

a corpsman. To my surprise he asked, "Do you have any preference?" (The Services had a reputation for not assigning enlisted men to positions for which they were qualified or interested.) In college, of the premedical subjects, only psychology had caught my fancy, so I said I would like to be assigned to a psychiatric ward. Again to my surprise, I was! The corpsman handed me a tiny chit of paper with my name at the top and "Ward 77B" written at the bottom. Three weeks later I would be reassigned to laundry duty—fulfilling my earlier suspicion—but not before those brief three weeks on the psych ward proved memorable.

Ward 77B held mostly ambulatory patients, primarily men who had returned from duty in the Pacific with mental diagnoses. My primary duties included cleaning, the occasional changing of bedpans, chatting with patients, and reporting anything untoward to the doctors. An older senior physician-psychiatrist had an office on the ward, but I rarely saw him. Most of my interaction was with the young—very young— physicians there as interns. During the war most medical schools were in session continuously, allowing for no break in between years, so four years of study were compressed into thirty-six calendar months. Consequently, the graduates—called "three year wonders"—were much younger than they should have been. One tall skinny man with glasses smoked a pipe, probably more so for the effect of trying to look older and wiser, than for actual enjoyment.

The patients on the ward offered me my first look at how unpredictable and thought-provoking the practice of medicine could be. One of my earliest experiences involved a man who looked and acted like a robot. Technically he was catatonic, but "zombie" was always the word that came to mind. Being new on the ward, I had no idea how he had become this way, nor how his doctors were treating him. One morning I came in to find him completely transformed. He was cheery, even laughing, talking volubly and clearly. He told me he had received a letter from his wife, whom he thought had deserted him while he was overseas, telling him she still loved him. Apparently she was the cure he needed! I was pleased and impressed. I also remember thinking this would allow for a good opportunity to have a serious discussion with the senior doctor and impress him with my intelligence. I managed to catch him, and when I described my observations, all he said was "Hmmm." Whether the patient had hysteria, was malingering, or had some variant of what we now call post-traumatic stress disorder, I will never know. But I do understand such distinctions may be quite difficult to determine still today.

One Saturday evening, while I was on duty, one of the patients returned from liberty with shaking chills and a high spiking fever. He told me "Doc, (the standard term of reference for corpsmen), my malaria is back." Malaria was a common disease in the South Pacific, and its prevention and treatment were not always effective—one form, in particular, was known to be prone to frequent relapse. I phoned the doctor on call, expecting he would tell me to give the man quinine to treat the infection, and thereby, relieve his fever. But instead he said, "Call the lab and order a thick and thin blood smear promptly." The patient sat there shaking violently with teeth-chattering, bone-shattering chills. One of the three-year wonders came to the ward with pipe in mouth and said we simply had to wait for the blood smear results to confirm the diagnosis. Finally, after a lengthy waiting period, the man's blood was drawn, finally the smear examined, finally the diagnosis established, and finally treatment begun. To my mind, making the patient wait all that time seemed insufferable.

This was my first experience with the struggle physicians may feel between compassion and rational analysis. The desire to do something quickly in an effort to relieve suffering and, in some cases, to save a life, frequently conflicts with the need to first establish the evidence required to determine the correct course of action. That night on the ward, I understood the issue intellectually, but remained upset. It would certainly not be the last time I was to face this kind of struggle, often in more complex situations. I remain convinced that no absolute principle to deal with such conflict exists; each event must be dealt with on its own merits. And to this day I wonder whether or not we should have treated the malaria patient more promptly.

On another long night, I was assigned as a special nursing assistant to sit and care for an older man dying of kidney failure. Remember this was long before the days of dialysis and transplantation. The man

3

was thin, bone dry, and comatose. His parched lips hung limply on his open mouth. I settled in at his bedside, expecting a relatively easy night. Suddenly I listened: was he breathing? He's not breathing! But before I could alert someone, I heard him take a short shallow breath followed by another louder, longer breath. His breathing continued and expanded until each breath was horribly loud, long and deep. Then, once again, his breathing stopped abruptly, completely. My fear returned until his breathing started up again, only to repeat the same terrifying pattern. I called the nurse and, despite my attempt to sound calm, my shaky voice gave away my growing anxiety. "Oh," she said, quite casually, "that's Cheyne-Stokes respiration. They do that." Indeed, "they"—terminal patients with many conditions—do. It was a frightful experience with what other physicians termed "Cheyne-Stoking." And it surely wouldn't be my last.

All told, I spent eight months at Oak Knoll during 1944 when shiploads of wounded men arrived from Saipan, Tinian and elsewhere in the South Pacific. My other assignments ranged from laundry service to public relations but never again involved direct patient care. So my pharmacist's mate medical experience was limited to those first fascinating three weeks, which, nonetheless, made for some indelible impressions.

In December 1944, to my great pleasure and relief, the Navy ordered me to attend the University of Illinois Medical School in Chicago. I was thrilled to report—in uniform—to the University, eager to begin the next phase of my medical education.

Medical School

One swallow does not a summer make

My first two years of school, characteristic of medical education at the time, had been spent almost entirely in lecture halls and laboratories, with minimal exposure to actual patients. In the third year lectures continued, but most of our time was now spent on the wards and in the clinics, first as observers and then as participants in the actual practice of medicine. It was a totally different and much more pleasurable and exciting world. Our Pediatric professors, Henry Poncher and Julius Richmond, were great lecturers; it seemed as if the relevant body of knowledge of Pediatrics was logical and all-encompassing. I liked the prospect of watching healthy infants and children grow, and participating in their development. At one well baby clinic located out in farm country, a grizzled couple in their forties had brought in their ten-month old for a routine evaluation. The boy, broad and firm, had more than tripled his birth weight. He sat bolt upright on his father's lap, looking like the offensive tackle I was certain he would turn out to be. Checking on diet, I asked, "What does he eat?"

The father was curt, as if the answer was obvious: "He eats what we eat." And thus I learned about the nutrition of farm children! It is no surprise that I was drawn to Pediatrics and envisioned a career as a pediatrician.

Then I went to work on the Pediatric wards. Sick children, and the feelings they aroused, differed greatly from healthy children. I remember admitting Jimmy, a lively eight-year-old boy. The pain in his legs suggested he had acute rheumatic fever, a sequela of strep throat, and a common disease in children and young adults then. A blood count, however, revealed deadly leukemia, a disease not yet curable, as it is today. Only a year before, when Jimmy had had his appendix removed, his blood count had been normal. How tragic for him, for his family! Having to deal with such devastating scenarios as a family losing a child suddenly made Pediatrics much less attractive.

Towards the end of that rotation I admitted a new patient I'll call Stella Mae. She was ten, a pretty little girl with blond curls. She, too, had leukemia, as I noted to my distress. When I leafed through her records, I found that she had also had her appendix removed, two years previously. An ironic coincidence!

Later that year on Internal Medicine, I cared for a man in his seventies, who also had been diagnosed with chronic leukemia. And there again, his records showed him to have had his appendix removed as a young man. Three cases of leukemia, three prior appendectomies. Could I be on to something?

I thought about it: the appendix is located at the terminus of the small bowel, an area full of lymphatic tissue. Indeed, the appendix itself usually contains lymphoid follicles. Could their removal have stimulated the rest of the body to over-produce those cells, resulting in leukemia? I went to the library to research further, but I could not find anything which noted the association. I realized three cases were but a few, but I, nevertheless, felt the thrill of having possibly stumbled upon a seminal discovery.

But my excitement was short-lived. My next leukemia patient had his appendix intact, as did the multiple others whose charts I reviewed. My little serendipitous cluster had represented nothing more than pure coincidence. It was an object lesson of the risk of jumping, even tentatively, to conclusions. One swallow does not a summer make.

Bedside Manner

Remember "bedside manner?" It was once considered the most essential characteristic of the successful practitioner. It had nothing to do with scientific or technical competence; it seemed to refer to personal charm accompanied by an exudation of self-confidence, necessary before the days of patient autonomy. A doctor's paternalistic decisions, calmly and succinctly presented, were to be accepted without question. Compassion, even sympathy, were not only unnecessary, they were frowned upon. In those days, the ideal physician was one who possessed "Aequinimitas"—equanimity: control and objectivity in the face of stressful situations. A patient's concerns and conditions were not to provoke any kind of emotional response from the ideal physician. As graduating medical students in 1948, we had all been given a copy of Sir William Osler's book, *Aequinimitas*; it portrayed the ideal towards which we were to strive.

Two incidents early in my training exemplify my struggle towards this ideal. The first occurred early in my third year of medical school. I was one among a group of students in an outpatient nose and throat clinic. We were asked to gather around and observe a patient, a small elderly woman, who sat in a chair wearing a threadbare coat lined with a scraggly fur; a small hat sat awry on a head of stringy hair. I noticed her eyes were tearing, and she made little noises resembling something between a whine and a whimper. We were told she had been treated for cancer of the mouth. All her teeth had been removed before the tumor had been irradiated; now, having returned to the clinic for a follow-up exam, the woman had a large ulcerated growth on the floor of her mouth, indicating a probable recurrence of the cancer. She was not named, nor was she introduced to us; the professor held her mouth open with a retractor the entire time he told us her story. He said she needed a biopsy to confirm the tumor recurrence. And then, to our great surprise, particularly mine, he turned to me, held out a biopsy forceps and said, "Here, take a bite of it with this."

A bewildering moment followed. I took the forceps. The woman looked at me, and I at her. She continued to whimper. The poor thing!

My emotions raced between horror, pity, and dread of having to "take a bite of it." The entire experience seemed bizarre, as if I were in some other universe. I had no prior experience with biopsy forceps, nor with *any* interventional procedure. Surely I would do something incorrectly and cause her great pain. I just wasn't ready for this. Finally I said, "I can't do it," and handed the forceps back to the professor. The forceps were handed over to another student, who boldly did as instructed, and soon it was over.

I was terribly embarrassed, sure that my classmates now considered me a sort of wimp, incompetent, unable to act like a professional, not fit for the practice of medicine. And I felt as though they may well have been right. Nobody said anything, but I knew the underlying doubt was in their minds, as well as my own.

The incident triggered some serious self-examination: was I choosing the right profession? Did I have what it took to be a competent physician? Moments of self-doubt can eventually lead to building inner strength and determination. I gained more training and proceeded to hone my technical skills throughout the rest of the year, but the experience of that first exposure became an indelible memory.

I offer here a second seminal, and quite contrasting, experience, one that occurred during my internship. I was then involved socially with a non-medical group of people, whose lifestyles and attitudes differed from mine. Relationships were volatile. One of the young women in the group—whom I was feeling hostile towards—approached me when I was working in the outpatient department. Her menstrual period was delayed; she feared she might be pregnant. Was there anything I could do? Those were days before simple pregnancy tests. However, the substance prostigmine, a smooth muscle stimulant, was believed to increase blood flow to the uterus. If a woman were pregnant, no harm would ensue from its use; but if her period was simply delayed, an intramuscular injection of prostigmine would bring the period on.

I reacted to her story coldly, due to my negative feelings towards her. I took her into a cubicle and, with no attempt at minimizing the distress she might have felt, jabbed the injection into her buttock. I sent her on her way with no guilt about my callous behavior.

A few days later word reached me from another member of the group: not only had her period come on, but I was reported to have behaved admirably in the most professional manner possible! Everyone was impressed with behavior I deemed cold and heartless.

The passage of time has helped me reevaluate both these early sophomoric occurrences. A bit ashamed of myself for my actions in the second case, I am delighted to believe that no one today would react to such insensitive behavior as positive. Surely I would be criticized for inadequate interpersonal skills, for lacking, at the very least, sympathy—even equanimity.

I have also reinterpreted my reluctance to biopsy the elderly woman's cancer in the first case. Yes, fear and inexperience led to my inaction. But I also know that I found the indignity of the entire situation abhorrent, the totally impersonal manner of the surgeon towards another human being, upsetting. I am proud of my empathetic reaction to that poor woman.

How different the situation is today! The patient is a partner; in fact, the patient is in charge. We physicians must sharpen our communication skills; we need to understand, accept and sympathize with our patients' feelings and reactions. We offer our recommendations as multiple options, the choice to be made by the patient. If asked, as is still not rare, "Well, what would you do, doctor, if you were me," we must explain gently that we are not they, and that a decision that might fulfill our needs might by very different from theirs. On the other hand, our experience as physicians gives us a broad and knowledgeable view of the possible outcomes and risks, even while recognizing that each person's situation differs. Physicians have abdicated their paternalistic positions, not always, I think, to the benefit of the patient. Whether or not we call it "bedside manner" today, the physician's demeanor requires a happy medium between paternalism, empathy and respect for patient autonomy.

A *"Classic"* Case

I was a new internal medicine clerk on the ward at Cook County Hospital. The patient, Otto Goetz, was a middle aged man, very dapper, with a short mustache, clearly a cut above the usual County clientele. He was European, in fact Austrian, and the early life he described was that of a bon vivant, complete with wine, women and song. His complaint was difficulty walking. When he walked, his feet were wide apart; he looked quite unstable. As we watched him come down the hospital corridor, all the medical students and house officers nodded in recognition of this absolutely classic presentation of a so-called *tabetic gait*—a typical end result of *tabes dorsalis*, a late nervous system complication of syphilis.

When I had taken this man's history, I learned of his fond memories of Vienna. We spoke about music and the opera there before the war, about which I knew a bit. He enjoyed the nostalgia, and the discussion made for good rapport between us. But then, as part of his "work-up," I performed a spinal tap on him—my first—and the procedure proved difficult due to my inexperience. It left him angry and in some pain—so much for doctor-patient relations.

The bigger medical lesson for me and everyone else involved, however, was that his syphilis tests all came back negative! And so much for apparently "classic" cases. It took further investigation to finally determine the correct diagnosis: pernicious anemia. Its serious neurologic complications affect the same zone of the spinal cord as does syphilis. What is classic, in fact, is that it is often mistaken for syphilis, since the presentation and resulting gait are similar in both diseases. Ironically, pernicious anemia is about as common in Northern Europeans as syphilis had been in the time of Austrian-born Schubert, of whom this patient was a great admirer.

First, Do No Harm

One afternoon early in my Medicine clerkship I admitted a young black man named Eddie Blackstone. He was unusual in many respects, one of which was that he was taller than I (and I stand 6'3"). Eighteen years old, thin, light-skinned, handsome, Eddie had a eunuchoid build and features. His reason for admission was also unusual. He had had hepatitis, an inflammation of the liver probably due to a virus, some weeks before. During hospitalization for it, he had undergone a new procedure: a sample of his liver had been taken via a biopsy needle inserted through his skin. This was the first I had heard of this type of procedure. Two separate research aspects were under study: one, experience with the biopsy itself, and second, study of the tissue characteristics of hepatitis. In fact, Eddie had already undergone two such biopsies during his earlier hospitalization, the first shortly after his admission, the second just before his discharge, as his hepatitis was subsiding. His liver had been enlarged, and the biopsies had been taken directly from it, as it extended below his rib cage.

Eddie was now being admitted for a third biopsy, in the recovery and, perhaps, healed phase of the hepatitis. Exactly what he had been told about the reasons for his third biopsy and the risks involved was unknown to me. What was clear was that no benefit would accrue to Eddie himself from the procedure; it was for the purpose of further research. The days of informed consent regarding research procedures were far in the future, so I doubt the discussion with him about it had been extensive. I do not even recall if a signed consent for the procedure had been obtained. No matter. Late in the afternoon the research team arrived on the ward. Eddie's liver had regressed to its normal size; it no longer could be felt extending below the rib cage—a good sign, indicating that Eddie's hepatitis was, indeed, resolving. Since the liver was now smaller, the biopsy was, therefore, performed from the side with the needle being inserted between two of his ribs, through the intercostal space.

We all understood the anatomy of the intercostal space well. We had to—fluid effusions around the lungs were commonly tapped and the fluid removed via needles inserted between the ribs into the pleural space. We knew the intercostal arteries and veins accompanied the ribs along their lower margins; we were careful to insert our needles into the intercostal space just above the top of the lower rib.

The needles used to tap pleural fluid were generally quite thin in caliber, as are the liver biopsy needles in use today. But the liver biopsy needle used that day on Eddie was not. It was a wide contraption with two prongs which separated as they entered the liver; an outer sheath was then passed over the prongs to trap a piece of tissue, which was then extracted for the biopsy.

The liver research team performed the biopsy, applied a bandage, and left the ward. Eddie returned to his bed on the ward to recuperate.

Early that evening, after I had completed my work and was about to leave, I checked on Eddie. He had no pain, but he complained of some difficulty breathing. In fact, his breathing had become rapid, and he looked pale. I examined him. I percussed over the area where the biopsy had been performed. The sound seemed dull to me in contrast to the resonant sound I elicited when my fingers tapped the normal air filled zones over lung. And I could not hear strong breath sounds in the same zone. These two findings probably indicated a fluid collection. I called the intern on the service, who confirmed my findings. He suggested that an intercostal vessel, probably the artery, had perhaps been damaged by the biopsy with resultant bleeding into the chest. He called the thoracic surgeons to come evaluate Blackstone and, presumably, to operate and tie off the bleeding vessel. He reassured me, and I left the ward.

When I returned in the morning, Eddie was not there, but his chart still was. What I read filled me with horror: a notation made at each hour of the night, from 8:00 p.m. until 4:00 a.m., stated "awaiting thoracic surgery." The nurses' notes described Eddie's increasing difficulty with breathing. At 4:15 a.m. he had been pronounced dead.

I could not believe it. I could not believe this vital healthy youth was dead. I could not believe the liver research team had not returned to the ward to check him. I could not believe the surgeons, presumably occupied elsewhere, had never arrived. We, the medical team, had been responsible for this fatal complication. My horror and shock at such an injustice turned into furious indignation at the medical team, myself included. Was this what the practice of medicine was like? Had it happened because we were in a County Hospital? Had Eddie's race been a factor? How could something like this have occurred—with me as a participant—in this golden age of medicine?

Hippocrates, who lived in the fifth and fourth centuries BCE, is considered the father of Western medicine. Probably his most famous aphorism is "First, Do No Harm." We...*I*...miserably failed Eddie in this regard. The experience had an immense impact on me and my nascent medical career. It was a rude awakening to see the fallibility of the system. My sense of guilt was accompanied by an increased feeling of responsibility. I resolved to always remember the lessons that I learned from Eddie in an attempt to prevent similar occurrences in the future. Looking back, I hope I have done so. I welcomed the establishment of informed consent when finally introduced decades later. Yet to this day I shudder when I think of Eddie Blackstone and those hard lessons learned.

Mantle of Power

My third year of medical school was grueling. I spent time on all the major clinical services, applying the facts and principles learned from textbooks and lectures to living, breathing patients. The hours were long, the stresses great, the attitudes and techniques difficult to master. But it was all worth it: I could feel myself transitioning from student towards physician.

The fourth year seemed easier, more relaxed, as I was more confident in my knowledge and skills. On my clinical rotations I was now more of a participant, rather than an observer and student.

On the surgical service at the Illinois University Hospital, then called R&E—the Research and Educational Hospital—I admitted Peter Rustin to the inpatient service. He was having some difficulty swallowing. As an outpatient, a barium swallow—a test to determine the cause of painful swallowing—had revealed an obstruction in his lower esophagus, strongly suggesting a cancer there. He was admitted for surgical exploration.

Rustin was a tall, thin, sixtyish, pleasant black man. When I asked him about his symptoms, he said the major thing bothering him was "water brash." This was a new phrase to me, and he seemed impatient with my lack of knowledge of the term. I pushed him to explain it further, and he did. I concluded he was describing fluid, perhaps acid, regurgitation from his "stomach" into his mouth. Its recent increase would surely be compatible with possible obstruction in his esophagus. He had lost some weight, but otherwise, his "review of systems"—questions asked of the patient to determine any possible abnormalities elsewhere in the body— revealed nothing unusual.

I proceeded to the physical exam. His heart and lungs were fine; I felt no abnormal lymph nodes in his neck or elsewhere. I paid special attention to his abdomen, and, except for its thinness, found nothing abnormal. This was true for the rest of his body as well. I found nothing to suggest any other illness or spread of the tumor. Nothing, that is, until I came to the routine neurologic exam. When stimulated by my reflex hammer, the reflexes in Rustin's left arm seem more active than those on the right. When I came to his legs, my impression was confirmed: his left knee jerk was clearly greater than his right. The same was true for the ankle jerk. And when I scratched the sole of his left foot, his big toe turned upwards, instead of down, as had the right. This positive Babinski reflex, along with my other findings, suggested an abnormality in the right side of the brain, in his right cerebral cortex. I asked him again about symptoms, about anything in the past that might account for these changes. He claimed he had none.

The diagnosis seemed straightforward to me. The cancer had probably spread to his brain, in which case, surgery on the esophagus would do little to cure him. I completed my write-up, concluding with my diagnosis: *carcinoma of the esophagus with metastasis to the right cerebral hemisphere.*

When I had been a third-year student, it was customary to list all other possible diagnoses, whether common or rare, that could account for a patient's condition. Now, as a senior, I felt such a listing unnecessary. Yes, there existed other possibilities, but I felt confident in my diagnosis.

The next time I came to the ward Rustin was gone. I found the surgery resident: where was he? "We discharged him. That was a good pick-up by you—saved him an unnecessary operation." And that was that.

I was amazed and a bit appalled. I could not believe I—a fourth-year med student—had acquired such power. My physical exam and diagnosis had been accepted completely. I had directly influenced a patient's care and life just like that. I assumed the resident had verified my physical findings, yet no other confirmatory studies had been done, even though there existed other possibilities for his condition: a prior stroke, a previous brain injury—many other reasons in addition to my one cavalier diagnosis of a metastasis. Without any further study, without any confirmation, was such confidence in my findings and diagnostic ability reasonable? My power to solely determine a patient's treatment (or lack thereof) seemed exorbitant, shockingly excessive.

It was a stunning lesson for me. The physician's power is immense—a few poorly chosen words can carry life and death implications. I resolved to be more careful in my pontifical pronouncements, now realizing for the first time that I was wearing the mantle of power—it having been slipped over my shoulders without my knowledge—for good or for ill.

Internship

In Medical School I was in many respects less attentive to planning a
medical career than I should have been. By the end of my junior year
I felt as if I knew just about all there was to know, which made my senior
year seem redundant. Unlike today, when one starts specialty training
immediately after medical school, then entirely separate "rotating"
internships were the norm, after which one could begin general practice
or go on to residency. Applications were completed towards the middle
of the senior year.

I applied to four hospitals, feeling certain that, given my excellent
academic record and class ranking, I would get into all of them. Two
were in Chicago: Cook County and the University of Illinois Hospital
(called R & E, Research and Education); the third one, which I
considered my "backup," was Kings County Hospital in Brooklyn.
Almost by happenstance, I decided to apply to a fourth—Mt. Sinai—
after overhearing one of my classmates talk about Mt. Sinai as one of
the top places to go. As I had a strong desire to return to New York, I
applied there as well.

I received invitations to interview at Cook County Hospital and Mt.
Sinai. Only later did I learn that it was rare for Sinai even to consider
anyone other than graduates of the New York medical schools. My
interview at Cook County turned out to be rather unmemorable, as it

consisted of the standard 'Why have you decided to apply to Cook County, and why do you want to pursue a career in medicine' sort of questions. I assumed I aced it, no problem. That left the Mt. Sinai interview.

Mt. Sinai was beautifully located, on Fifth Avenue and 100th St., across from Central Park. The interview took place in a distinguished wood-lined board room. Seated, were half a dozen men, but the only person I remember was Dr. Isidore Snapper, one of the Medicine chiefs, who conducted the interview. He wasted no time. "Tell me about bronchiectasis" (a lung disease), he said. In my response, I mentioned clubbing, a change in the fingertips, which is one sign of bronchiectasis. "Tell me about clubbing," he said. I did. "And why do people get it?" I mentioned low blood oxygen. "But some people with clubbing don't have that," he challenged. The interview went on like this for over an hour. He wove an intellectual tapestry between isolated findings, connecting and disconnecting, in an immensely exciting way. I had never experienced anything like it in medical school. When that interview was over, I walked back out onto Fifth Avenue. It was a beautiful spring day. And I wanted that internship at Mt. Sinai more than I had ever wanted anything.

To my everlasting surprise, I was not accepted for internship at either Cook County or Kings County. I was accepted at R & E, and I was offered an alternate position at Mt. Sinai, which meant someone else had to drop out first before a formal offer would be extended to me. The likelihood of that happening was slim. R & E wanted my response immediately, but I continued to put them off for a few days, while I anxiously awaited the call from Mt. Sinai. It finally came. They offered me a position, and I said yes on the spot.

Upon graduation, having been accepted at one of the top hospitals, I smugly figured that internship would be a year of simply firming up my already vast knowledge with some practical experience. I quickly discovered that nothing about that year would be simple, and that I still had quite a lot to learn.

Listen to the Patient!

Benjamin Rosenberg was one of my first patients on Internal Medicine during my internship. Rosenberg, a Jewish man about sixty-five, had peripheral vascular disease—a hardening of the arteries in his legs which had led to poor circulation. When he was admitted he also suffered from additional problems: early kidney failure and elevated blood pressure. We discovered he was diabetic. Despite his physical challenges, Rosenberg continued to be an active man, nevertheless, and being a gregarious fellow, he would make daily rounds in his wheel chair visiting the other patients on the ward.

In those days the medicine ward was an open ward with forty beds, with only a few private rooms in the rear. When a patient on the ward became acutely ill, we would wheel the bed into one of the rear rooms. Also, if someone should die on the ward, instead of pronouncing him dead in front of the other patients (an uncomfortable situation for all), we would slap an oxygen mask on the face, take the patient to the rear, and make the pronouncement there. This had happened to Frank Meinert, an elderly cardiac patient who was a friend of Rosenberg's. Afterwards, Rosenberg was overheard saying, "They take them to the back, but when I go visit, they're not there! Where do they go?" I don't think he ever figured it out.

Rosenberg's poor circulation soon led to gangrene of the toes on one of his feet. This development was not entirely unexpected, but what was unusual was that his toes became infected. Ben's temperature rose, and the infection began to spread up his leg. We started penicillin (broader spectrum antibiotics were not yet available) but it made little difference. His blood sugar began to rise precipitously. Sugar then spilled over into his urine, which was increasing in volume. With this uncontrolled infection the biggest fear was that he might progress to diabetic acidosis, a very serious complication. To help stabilize him, I quickly started an intravenous infusion of fluid, while our team and attending physicians evaluated the situation. It was decided Rosenberg needed insulin to control the worsening of his diabetes. It was my job to inform him of this rather standard procedure. To my surprise, Ben replied, "Dr. Green, don't give me insulin. If you give me insulin, I will die."

19

My internship was in the days of paternalistic medicine; the principle *Doctor knows best* was firmly established, so it was rare that a patient would reject a doctor's recommendation or refuse planned therapy. I reassured Mr. Rosenberg. "Don't be silly, Ben," I said, "the amount of insulin I will give you will be small; I will also add glucose—sugar—to your IV, so there will surely be no problem with excess insulin."

Rosenberg remained resolute, stating, "No, Dr. Green, don't do it. Insulin will kill me." He and I went back and forth a bit. I could not learn the source of his unreasonable fear, and the indication for insulin was crystal clear. I calmly insisted and added the glucose to the IV. Then I added the insulin. All the while, Rosenberg was aware of my actions. I reassured him again; all was going well. Half an hour later it was Benjamin Rosenberg who died and whom we wheeled to the back room.

"Listen to the Patient" is a medical aphorism I have taught many times in lectures and workshops over the years. The admonition clearly refers to paying careful attention to the patient's history; the second meaning emphasizes the importance of the physical examination of the chest. The phrase, however, also has a third, quite literal meaning, as taught to me that day by Benjamin Rosenberg, one that I will never forget.

Today it is rare that a physician would insist on proceeding, if a patient so insistently refuses a procedure and cannot be convinced otherwise. The intervention simply would not proceed.

Routines, routines

One day a man named Willie Russell was admitted to my ward. In his forties, solidly built, Willie claimed good health until the prior week. He had caught a bad cold, which promptly affected his lungs. He got a prescription for a sulfa drug, and took it. Three days later he noticed a diminution in his urine output, which rapidly progressed to a total absence of urination. His physical exam was entirely normal; he looked like a vigorous, healthy man. To me, the diagnosis was straightforward:

he had had a serious kidney reaction to the sulfa drug, and his poisoned kidneys had shut down. The biggest question was how to proceed. Did we restrict fluids until his kidneys recovered spontaneously, or did we push fluids, in the hope that extra volume would help force urine flow? The Urology division was consulted. (An old memory: we filled out a small chit of paper, marked it PSNOC—please see note on chart—and put it in the Urology mailbox.)

The Urology resident, a handsome young man named Harold Lear, came to see Willie. After reviewing the case, he scheduled a cystoscopy—a procedure in which the bladder is examined via a lighted tube placed into the urethra. I objected; the bladder was not enlarged by physical exam; surely the diagnosis was clear, and this uncomfortable procedure unnecessary. Lear addressed me calmly and thoughtfully, (in contrast to the peremptory manner I was accustomed to from many surgeons) saying, "Yes, the sulfa was the likely culprit, but one just had to be sure that something, such as an enlarged prostate gland, wasn't obstructing the flow of urine." This was the proper routine, and the procedure was really quite simple. If obstruction did exist, the possibility of missing it would be tragic. (Today an ultrasound of the abdomen, which is not invasive, would be the first procedure performed, based on the same principle.)

Before this, I had found the constant demand for routine procedure by doctors to be a sign of uncompromising rigidity. That day, Lear's insistence on customary procedure convinced me otherwise. To everyone's surprise, perhaps even Lear's, a cancer was discovered inside Willie's bladder that had spread to block the entrance of both ureters, the tubes that connect the kidneys to the bladder.

Willie had had no symptoms at all prior to the acute urinary shutdown. Rigidity and routine, I learned from Harold Lear, have little in common other than the initial letter "r."

I later was privileged to spend a month on Urology with Hal Lear, from whom I learned a great deal. I saw no special cases there, but actually, one common experience was immensely satisfying. As a big medical diagnostician-to-be, I prided myself on solving complex problems; yet I rarely brought as much relief to any patient than I did when I passed urinary catheters on men whose urination had been blocked for one reason or another—men with acute urinary retention.

In those days the common operation for an enlarged prostate was done in two stages: in the first, a tube was placed into the bladder to decompress it; the prostate was removed in the second stage. The tube was connected to a large bottle to collect the urine. The ward was full of men walking around, holding their bottles while waiting for their second operation. We interns sang an irreverent song: "Around, the ward, they haul their jugs of urine, And to those bottles they maritally cling"; it concluded with "The biggest of collections is sure to win a prize, though the amount that it can piddle is no function of its size." This situation was a source of amusement for us interns.

Harold Lear enjoyed a distinguished medical and surgical career. He died, sadly, at much too young an age of heart disease. He is the subject of *Heart-sounds*, a moving biography written by his wife, Martha Weinman Lear.

All the World Over

'There are more things in heaven and earth, Horatio,
Than are dreamt of in your philosophy.'

Hamlet

Esmerelda was a beautiful young woman with chiseled features and light reddish hair. Her fair skin made it hard to believe she was from the mountains and not the cities of Peru, because one would have assumed she was Castilian rather than native Indian in ethnicity. And perhaps she was, with a family history long lost. She apparently basically spoke Spanish, but with a dialect our local Puerto Rican Spanish translator found difficult to understand. Her illness was puzzling, and our approach to it influenced, I am certain, by the language barrier. Esmerelda had been ill for some months. Her primary complaint was diffuse abdominal pain and fever, yet by outward appearances, she looked fairly well. She lay placidly in bed, often smiling and never complaining. We performed the various gastrointestinal studies available to us at the time; they were all unrevealing. On physical examination, however, her belly was a bit more prominent than her chest and extremities, as if it were swollen. Indeed, it had a firm, but not hard consistency, feeling almost "doughy." Physicians reading this will recognize the word, as it is commonly used to describe the feel of an abdominal wall over tuberculous inflammation with a fluid collection in the peritoneal space (the peritoneum is the membrane that lines the wall of the abdomen), so it seemed Esmerelda had tuberculous peritonitis. Indeed, there was something about her that reminded me of Henry Matthews, another patient I had seen when I was a medical student, who had also suffered from this form of tuberculosis.

We tapped her abdomen and sent a small amount of fluid to the laboratory for study. Dr. Snapper, the Chief of the Service, examined her and concurred in the diagnosis. "And how do you treat TB peritonitis?" he asked us. Several of us suggested that streptomycin, a recently discovered antibiotic, would help. Another one of the residents said he had read that injection of air into the peritoneal space could also be helpful. "No," said Dr. Snapper. He offered a bizarre recommendation: "You go to the operating room, get some of the thick jellied soap the surgeons use to scrub their hands, and you smear it all over the abdomen; then you cover it all with coarse paper towels." It seemed a strange remedy, but in those days you didn't argue with the Chief. Off to the operating room I went, retrieved the soap and proceeded as instructed. As I smeared the material on Esmeralda's abdomen, a remarkable transformation took place: Esmerelda's demeanor completely changed, so that by the time I finished, she was noisily babbling in Spanish, waving her arms, flushed, excited in a manner totally unlike any of her previous behavior. An interpreter finally arrived. Esmerelda told us that as a little girl, high in the Andes, she had experienced a similar illness. Her grandmother had done exactly the same as I was now doing—she had smeared some sticky material on her belly and covered it with broad leaves—and Esmerelda had recovered!

We were all amazed. I think "my philosophy had not dreamt of the possibility" that somehow, both in the mountains of South America and in the knowledge base of a sophisticated European physician, a similar folk remedy had taken hold. This was long before the days of effective antituberculous chemotherapy and certainly before evidence-based medicine; if one had asked about the studies showing such jellied soap as a successful treatment, you would probably have been met with a blank stare. A list of remedies used in hope of gaining a cure would fill an entire volume by itself, and soap, acting as a counterirritant, offered as good an option as any.

In the days since Esmerelda I have been slower to dismiss folk remedies out of hand, although I remain skeptical about them until scientific studies provide some evidence of success and/or understanding of possible mechanisms. Yet the memory of Esmerelda's excitement that day as I rubbed the jelly on acts as a constant reminder to stay open to many of the complementary treatments and alternative medicines being tested today.

Blood Suckers

In 2006 the *New Yorker* magazine published an article by John Colapinto on leeches, entitled "Bloodsuckers." I was reminded of Mrs. Behrens, an elderly lady with pain and swelling due to chronic venous obstruction in one of her legs. And chronic it was: originally from South Africa, Behrens had sought help there, then in London, at a famous clinic elsewhere in the United States, and finally had come to Mt. Sinai. When I presented this history on rounds, Dr. Snapper smiled and said, "Why go to the branch offices when the main office is still open?" It was one of his favorite remarks.

Dr. Isidore Snapper was a tall man with a shiny bald pate and thick glasses. Originally from Holland, where he was a professor and involved in the care of the royal family, Snapper later was detailed by the Rockefeller foundation to the Peiping Medical College in China. He was taken prisoner when the Japanese invaded; later, in a prisoner exchange he came to this country and to Mt. Sinai.

Following the presentation on rounds Dr. Snapper discussed venous obstruction with us and asked us about treatment. We gave standard, fresh-from-medical-school answers: elevation of the leg, warm or cold compresses, tight stockings, various ointments, and others, most of which she had tried. Dr. Snapper was not satisfied. Such remedies would all be inadequate in a really recalcitrant case. His answer: apply a leech! Well, this would explain the supply of leeches we modern, newly-minted physicians had discovered in a tank one day on the ward. We learned that not only were leeches considered to be effective in such cases, but when leeches bit, they secreted a substance which was both a pain reliever and an anticoagulant.

But Dr. Snapper wasn't finished. What should we do if the leech wouldn't bite? Of course, we had absolutely no idea. "Apply a drop of Heineken's beer to the skin," said Dr. Snapper. "There has never been a leech born that can resist the taste of Heineken's." Mrs. Behrens improved and was discharged before we had the opportunity to test his pronouncement!

Mefiez Vous

Her name was Gussie Grossinger; she was admitted for workup of hyperthyroidism, an overactive thyroid gland. As the intern assigned I was the first to see her. She had had a prior admission to Mt Sinai, years before, and when I reviewed the record I saw that she had had a cardiac murmur, diagnosed as the diastolic murmur of mitral stenosis, sometimes a difficult one to hear. I listened to her, both before and after I saw the old chart, and I really didn't hear anything—at first. But, of course, the chart, presumably written by superb physicians of yore, recorded a murmur, so I listened and listened and, finally, I heard it, and recorded it in the write up of my physical exam.

Robert Wallerstein, later a prominent psychiatrist, was then my senior resident. After he had evaluated the patient he called me over, and we examined the patient together. He convinced me with no difficulty that there really was no murmur. I knew he understood the pressure I felt to hear it, and his intervention not only put the record right, but taught me the important and basic lesson to have more confidence in myself.

The next morning I presented the case to the attending physician. I

25

said that at first I had thought I heard a murmur, but then decided I had not. In a highly critical dismissive tone, the attending cut me off, saying there's no murmur, and we moved on to the rest of the case. I accepted the criticism because, of course, he was right and I was wrong.

The next day, Dr Snapper, the Chief, made rounds with his full entourage. Once again, I told the story of the murmur. Snapper, who was not regarded as a particularly strong cardiologist, listened carefully. He stood up. "Mefiez vous de la premiere impression," he said, "c'est toujours le meilleur." It was the first time I had heard him state one of his favorite aphorisms. *Beware of the first impression (that is, regard it highly); it is always the best.* "There *is* a murmur."

Later when we listened again, we were certain Snapper was wrong. Even though it was incorrect in Gussie's case, the lesson of "Mefiez vous" stayed with me and became a principle I used in my teaching for years.

Marshall

I admitted a young woman who was acutely ill with a sore throat, enlarged lymph nodes and abnormal tests of liver function. Infectious mononucleosis was the logical diagnosis, but on physical examination I was surprised to find that both her liver and her spleen were grossly enlarged, their palpable edges extending halfway down the abdomen towards her umbilicus. When, on rounds, I presented her case to Dr. Snapper, I said that I had never seen that degree of hepatic and splenic enlargement in mononucleosis. To which statement Dr. Snapper replied, "Marshall."

Should I know what that meant? I didn't, and so I asked. Dr. Snapper proceeded to tell a tale of an elderly American chess champion, named Marshall, who eventually travelled to Europe to play the even more elderly octogenarian European champion. To Marshall's astonishment, he was soundly beaten by the European. At a celebratory dinner after the contest, Marshall, still shaken, said that never in all his years had he experienced such a display of chess prowess. The European victor replied, "Well, you are young yet."

The point was well taken. When a physician says he has never seen a particular circumstance, implying a biologic rarity, it is most often a reflection on his or her own relative inexperience. It was remarkable how often, over the ensuing years, I heard young house officers use a similar phrase—to which I would respond, "Marshall," and repeat the story.

The Countess

I called her the Countess. I had good reason to. Maria Volkosky came from somewhere in central Europe; she would only say from "the Austrio-Hungarian Empire." Six feet tall with a stunning straight posture, she carried her excess weight beautifully. She wore a brightly colored turban around her upswept blondish hair, and she complemented it with a similarly colored robe. The Countess presented a remarkable sight, as she wandered around the ward, looking as if she was accepting obeisance from the other patients. What added to her striking appearance were the unusual color of her skin and the bright yellow color of the whites of her eyes: she was jaundiced.

I was the admitting intern. The story I elicited from her was not clear cut. Most of my questions about symptoms were answered rather vaguely with "Yes and No," "Sometimes," or "Not lately." As best I could piece it together, she had had recurrent episodes of pain in her belly, some minor, some major, for a long time—months, if not years. Her appetite came and went, with a random inability to tolerate some foods. Her weight fluctuated. More recently her urine was often dark. She couldn't tell me about the color of her stools, because "I never look." That first night, when I examined her, I found a deeply jaundiced woman. Her heart, lungs, extremities and lymph nodes were normal, but her abdomen was diffusely tender, without any true localization, although I could feel the liver edge. I felt a soft puffy density below the rib cage on the right; the next morning it was gone, and had probably represented stool. When I finished my exam, I sent off the appropriate laboratory tests.

Gall bladder disease—gall stones—seemed to me the most likely diagnosis. I postulated they were present in the gall bladder and were also obstructing the duct leading from the liver to the intestine, thus causing the jaundice. I also knew that the stereotypical gall bladder patient was "fair, fat, female and forty." Maria pretty much fit the bill. The next morning on rounds the team agreed with me.

In those days the laboratory tests available for the study of biliary tract and liver disease were limited. Surprise! The few tests we did have suggested the source of the trouble was her liver rather than the biliary tract, as I had thought. The team resolved into two parties: those whom I liked to call the "real doctors" supported my clinical diagnosis; the others, whom I derisively labeled "chemists," favored a sick liver, presumably due to hepatitis. Additional tests were conducted yet the exact cause remained a mystery. At one point, Maria's jaundice started to resolve, favoring the chemists; but then it relapsed, favoring the doctors' opinion that gall stones were obstructing the outflow of bile from the liver.

Dr. Snapper arrived for his professorial rounds. I repeated the history, and what had happened since. Perhaps not surprisingly, Dr. Snapper said, "Mefiez vous..." as I have described earlier in Gussie's case. "What you felt that first night was the gall bladder; Maria has a cancer of the pancreas or ampulla of Vater." He was referring to an old aphorism, Courvoisier's law: disease of the gall bladder inflames, scars and shrinks it; if new disease in the pancreas or collecting outlets blocks the bile flow, a previously healthy gall bladder will enlarge. If the obstruction is at the point where the bile enters the intestine, a structure termed the "ampulla of Vater," the obstruction can be intermittent, which would explain her waxing and waning jaundice. So now we had three possible causes : gall stones, sick liver and cancer of the pancreas or ampulla. The argument continued beyond the time I had left the Medicine service and rotated onto the Surgical service. Note, the differentiation between these three possibilities would be pretty straightforward today; it was not so then.

The Countess was eventually scheduled for exploratory surgery, and I was fortunate to be on the service to which she was transferred. I scrubbed in with Dr. Colp, the chief surgeon, and Dr. Klingenstein, his associate, as we prepared to explore the Countess's abdomen. While doing so, Dr. Colp said, "Green, what do you think we'll find?"

"Well, sir," I said, "I have thought this was gall stones from the start, and see no reason to change my mind."

"What do you think, Percy?" asked Dr. Colp.

"I think she had hepatitis, and now has hepatomatous (tumorous) transformation of the liver cells."

Colp then expressed his differing opinion: "This is cancer of the pancreas or the ampulla." We were not being competitive; the difference of opinion reflected the difficulty of the case.

Maria looked quite different, appearing at her most vulnerable as she lay stretched out on the operating table. Colp entered the abdomen rapidly and put in his hand. "Gall bladder, full of stones," he announced, "bile ducts, full of stones." The operation went well. Biopsies of the liver showed some damage from the now long standing obstruction, but it was clear the primary pathology had been the stones. Between thirty and forty beautiful brown sharply faceted stones were removed. We sent a few to the laboratory; I gave a few in a small container to Maria when she recovered. I kept the majority for myself in a large glass jar, as a reminder that, as stated in "Mefiez vous," first impressions often *are* correct, and that sometimes, at least, it is wise to stick with one's clinical impression when it conflicts with laboratory findings.

I am embarrassed

After the first four months of my rotating internship on Internal Medicine, my fifth month was in Admitting, which was both a walk-in clinic and the first stop for scheduled admissions. It was an exciting month due to the unpredictable nature of the clinic—we saw whomever walked in for whatever reason. The two attending physicians checked those patients whose admission had already been arranged. Both attendings were excellent. One of the reasons Mt. Sinai was a desirable internship was that the bedside teaching was oriented towards the interns, and this was true in Admitting as well. In those days, to obtain privileges to hospitalize your own patients at Mt. Sinai, a doctor had to donate some free time to the hospital. Few doctors were permitted to attend on the wards, so they usually attended in one clinic or another. All the old Jewish ladies used to say, "My doctor is Chief of the clinic at Mt. Sinai," and many of them were more or less correct.

One day Dr. Davidson, one of the attendings, instructed me as follows: "There's a lady in the next cubicle. I want you to go in and do a complete physical." "Complete" was a word with a not so hidden message. It usually meant, for either sex, a rectal exam. I went in, briefly said hello, did a quick general physical, finding nothing abnormal, and then slipped on a glove and performed a rectal exam. Her rectum was soft and wide, and on the posterior wall I could feel a very large, soft, slippery, fronded mass—obviously a rectal cancer. Yet the woman had been sent to the clinic for a completely different reason. I went out and discussed my findings with Dr. Davidson. He had already discovered the mass and wanted to impress upon me the importance of being thorough in my examinations. A lesson well learned.

In January I started on Surgery. Sinai had three surgical services: the Gastric Service headed by Dr. Ralph Colp; the Colon Service headed by Dr. John Garlock; and Arthur Touroff's Thoracic Service. While other conditions were admitted to any one of these services, each service represented that particular doctor's specialty area. I was assigned to Dr. Colp's service.

When I began the month, I of course inherited some patients whose hospitalizations had begun before my arrival. One was the very sad case of Mrs. Epstein, an elderly woman who had been admitted with a cancer of the middle (transverse) segment of the colon. She had been operated upon; although the cancer was apparently successfully removed, the line of sutures where the two segments of bowel had been reconnected had not held, with a resultant pathway or tract, called a fistula, from the colon to the skin. It required constant dressing (she leaked feces through it). In addition, post operatively it was discovered she had a second cancer in the rectum. Nothing could be done about it until she had sufficiently healed from the first operation. I tended to her dressings daily and gradually became more familiar with her.

One day I asked if I might examine her rectum, as I had not done so since I started on the service. "Oh, Dr. Green," she said, "you were one of the first ones to examine me." That couldn't be true. The poor lady was obviously confused. I did the examination. Unbelievably, it was the same rectum I had examined in the clinic two months before! The tragedy was that neither the physicians who had referred her in, nor the surgical team who admitted her, had adequately (if at all) checked her rectum before embarking on her colonic surgery, in spite of the rectal finding being clearly recorded in Dr. Davidson's admitting note! It was a troubling error of double omission on the part of the admitting surgeons on the ward.

There is an old joke about a patient who sees a doctor and says, "You remember me, doctor, I am Meyer, your patient with hemorrhoids."

The doctor says "I've never seen you before." They go back and forth like this, but eventually when the doctor examines the anus he says, "Oh, hello Meyer!"

Unfortunately, in Mrs. Epstein's case, the story was far from funny.

Once a Melanoma

Herbert Goldstein was bohemian. He was an artist living in Greenwich Village, who had a live-in woman who was not his wife, not something young interns expected in 1948. His chief complaint was very dramatic: he had severe intermittent cramping abdominal pain, which went in waves across his abdomen, he said, due to "worms." He had lost weight and was thin. That part of his story could be confirmed. During an attack, he would scream out loud in bloodcurdling fashion, and indeed, one could see subtle movements under his skin. We decided these were probably unusual peristaltic waves arising from his bowel. But why? The only other major abnormalities we noted were an enlarged liver, and an irregular scar on his back, which he said was from removal of a mole a decade earlier. We were stumped as to the cause of Herbert's periodic attacks.

Multiple studies were unrevealing, although his liver functions were slightly compromised. On rounds Dr. Snapper had an idea: obtain the microscopic slides of the mole. It might well have been a malignant melanoma. But that was years and years ago, we said, and what would that have to do with his "worms" anyway? No matter what it is, said Dr. Snapper, once you have a melanoma, any illness you get after that is going to be due to spread of the melanoma, no matter when it occurs (of course, an exaggeration of the truth). We interns were skeptical. When we obtained the slides we discovered that yes, in fact, a melanoma existed; yet this finding still didn't necessarily help provide a diagnosis.

Herbert's health continued to deteriorate. His pain worsened, his liver enlarged further. We needed answers. Since the liver was clearly the site of disease, a resident suggested doing a needle biopsy of it, according to Sutton's Law. (When Willie Sutton, the famous bank robber, was asked why he had chosen repetitively to rob banks, he replied, "Because that's where the money is.") This procedure was relatively new, and still considered rather risky. I was not strongly in favor of the biopsy, due to my previous experience with Eddie Blackstone in medical school, but the decision was not mine to make. The biopsy went off without incident or complication, and without revealing any new information. The microscopic examination indicated a normal liver.

Goldstein was finally transferred to the surgical service for laparotomy—exploratory abdominal surgery. Once he was opened, the answers were revealed with stunning clarity: his liver housed two giant "cannonball" masses of melanoma. The site of the biopsy had been in the normal tissue between the masses. The diagnosis was confirmed, but Herbert did not long survive the procedure.

At autopsy it was further revealed that the melanoma had spread to the submucosa (the inner lining) of the small bowel, among other locations. His bizarre attacks had been due to the resultant abnormal functioning of the bowel, in what were called recurrent minor intersuccessions. We learned from the literature that this was not a rare site for melanoma metastasis.

As Goldstein's death was postoperative, he was presented as a complication at surgical morbidity conference. One of the surgeons asked, "In view of the fact that the needle biopsy missed the tumor, and as it is a risky procedure, shouldn't patients just have open biopsies?"

To which Ralph Colp replied dryly, "The internists didn't do any worse than we did."

The "Once a melanoma..." lesson is an important one. In fact, in a common Sherlock Holmes type of quiz question, a patient with an enlarged liver is described whose only other significant feature is a glass eye. If you know that the retina is a site for melanoma, the answer is easy. Herbert Goldstein remains in my memory as a dramatic person with a dramatic illness, who taught me an equally dramatic lesson.

The lesson stood me in good stead. Many years later I was asked to consult on a man with widespread lung nodules strongly indicative of cancerous spread to the lungs. An extensive workup had been unrevealing. Accompanied by a large group of students and house officers, I greeted him, introduced myself and shook his hand. I noticed a scar on his right wrist. "What is that?"

"I had a mole removed many years ago," he responded.

Remembering Herbert's case years earlier, I immediately instructed, "Get the slides." The scar proved, on review, to have been a melanoma. My entourage learned three principles from this brief encounter: the power of observation, the courtesy and respect due all patients, and once a melanoma...

A not so careful choice of words

I was not especially interested in surgery, but I found my three months on the gastic surgical service instructive and pleasant due, in large part, to the colorful chief, Dr. Ralph Colp.

Colp was a tall muscular man, a ramrod straight figure with a military bearing. He had a big white mustache and graying hair and wore sport jackets with colorful contrasting patterned vests. Colp radiated vigor, not age. His aristocratic appearance belied his lower East Side upbringing, revealed only by his thick New York accent. His vigor extended to the operating room, where he was known to operate rapidly. His primary assistant, Dr. Percy Klingenstein, who was shorter and thinner than Colp, spoke with a similarly accented but clipped voice. Their contrasting appearances and staccato dialogue reminded one of a comic duo. Percy was considered something of a yes man to Ralph.

At our New Year's Eve intern show, just before I started on their service, we performed a skit in which Colp and Klingenstein were portrayed consulting with naive internists. The dialogue started with Colp and went something like this:

"What's the complaint?"

"Pain."

"Which side?"

"Right side."

"High or low?"

"High."

"Gall bladder. What's today?"

"Tuesday."

"We'll operate on Thursday. I want a red blood count, a white blood count, and a blue blood count. We'll present this patient at grand rounds in Technicolor."

"You want a blood chemistry?"

"Yeah, get one of dem."

Then, Ralph asks his sidekick, "What do you tink of this case, Poicy?"

Percy responds, "I tink like you tink, Ralph."

The week after I started on the gastric surgery ward, I attended my first surgical grand rounds. Colp presented the case of a woman upon whom he had operated for colonic obstruction. He had found a large inflammatory mass, probably from diverticulitis. As removal was impossible, the standard treatment would have been a colostomy, which would divert the stool stream until the inflammation in her colon had subsided. However, Colp had cared for the woman's brother some years previously. The man had had rectal cancer with a horrible experience with a colostomy and eventual death. Colp explained that he felt if the woman awoke and found he had performed a colostomy, no conversation would convince her that she, unlike her brother, would be all right. He had, therefore, closed without doing one. Then Colp turned to Klingenstein. "What do you tink, Percy?"

"Well, Ralph," said Percy, "at the last New Year's Eve jamboree they had a skit where they said I always agree with you. So I am glad you asked me that question, because I am afraid that in this case I can't agree with you, Ralph." We could hardly keep from laughing. In the midst of this exaggerated humor I learned an important lesson: Never be afraid to rely on my own judgment or state my own opinions, even if they differed from standard practice, or the opinion of others.

Colp liked me. He would often question me on rounds and in the operating room, and he liked my responses. I scrubbed with him often, my role usually limited to holding the retractors. During one operation, however, I almost succeeded in spoiling our good rapport. At that time the standard operation for chronic duodenal ulcer on our service was removal of a large part of the stomach, called a subtotal gastrectomy, originated by an earlier Sinai surgeon, A. A. Berg. Colp proudly claimed to hold the world's record for speed—26 minutes skin to skin (from incision to closure)—for the procedure. One day I was holding the retractors as Colp slashed away. He said, "Green, where'd you go to Medical School?"

"The University of Illinois, sir."

"Who's the head of surgery there?"

"Warren Cole, sir."

Colp promptly retorted, "Oh yeah, Cole—sourpuss, ain't he?"

Actually, Dr. Cole did have a continually dour expression, but he was revered by his surgical residents; I responded with some platitude about his personality not matching his demeanor. That piqued Colp's interest, "What kind of surgeon is he?"

As a medical student I had scrubbed with Cole on a complicated biliary tract case. He had worn his glasses low on his nose, made little tiny incisions, and taken a look at what he was doing after each tiny cut. So without thinking about it I said, "Well, sir, he's very meticulous."

"Meticulous!" shouted Colp. "Don't say that word to me! Whaddya mean, he's slow?"

I could see his face turning red behind his mask. "I'm *meticulous* too—I just don't tie off every goddamn skin bleeder!" He slammed down his scalpel, muttering "meticulous," and shouted, "Give me some clean drapes." The chief resident assisting him, David Orringer (the uncle of Mark Orringer, who is now head of Thoracic Surgery at the University of Michigan), started to undo the clips holding the very, very bloody drapes on the skin surrounding the open incision. "No, no, just bring me some clean ones!" By his response, I had clearly hit a nerve. Colp continued to mutter "meticulous," ignoring me throughout the rest of the operation.

Fortunately, my politically incorrect remark had no lasting ill effects. In fact, when I left the service, Colp offered me a prized surgical residency with him. My professional and financial future would have been assured—but a surgical career did not appeal to me.

Again!

Colp and his entire service were immensely proud of their record performing the major operation of subtotal gastrectomy. As well they should have been. When I started on service they had performed 286 consecutive procedures without a single death—truly a remarkable record. Then came Frank Buffalino, a middle aged Italian man, admitted for the procedure. Frank had a long history of problems with ulcer, including surgery for a perforated ulcer many years before. He sported a visible scar on his abdomen as a result.

One of the other senior attendings was the operating surgeon. To our surprise, on the operating table we found a prior gastroenterostomy—a diverting procedure—which clearly was nonfunctional, since it hadn't shown up in the preoperative x-rays. We "took it down,"—corrected it—did the gastrectomy as planned, and closed. While the surgery had gone well overall, it became immediately apparent within hours afterwards that Buffalino was in trouble. His belly was distended and we could not get his intestines to function properly. Finally, persistent vomiting and a precarious state forced us to re-operate a few days later, late one Saturday night. What we found was a mess. We were unable to determine exactly what was wrong, and therefore, were unable to correct it. Despondently, we closed the incision. I stayed with Buffalino through the night, constantly restarting his IV's, repositioning, reinserting tubes, and doing whatever needed doing to keep him functioning. The prognosis and his chances for survival were poor.

Early Sunday morning the surgeon arrived for rounds and, with a big smile on his face, said, "Hey, it's really okay, because the series record is just for patients having their first major procedure, and Buffalino already had a gastroenterostomy, so he won't count!"

I was shocked and appalled at such a heartless statement. I unleashed my fury on him: "Okay, then take out the IV! Pull out the tubes, because it doesn't really matter!" The surgeon looked as if he was going to tear me apart, but one of the residents calmed him—and me—down, and everyone moved on. Somehow, some way, Buffalino gradually recovered—a testament to his will to live—and he was eventually discharged. I was proud my concern for a human life was greater than their track record. But it was another lesson for me regarding my need to think before I spoke, one I have not always observed.

And once more

Despite the unremitting stress of the surgery rotation, and the quotidian exposure to issues of life and death, occasional moments of levity sometimes offered welcome relief.

An intern's duties on any surgical service were pretty straightforward. Histories and physicals, scrubbing and holding retractors for major operations, blood drawing and IV starting, plus the opportunity to do minor surgical procedures oneself, under supervision. On a gastric service, however, one additional chore was the passing of tubes into the stomach. There was the Levin tube used for collecting gastric juice, and sometimes, feeding; the Rehfuss and Hollander tubes used for special tests; the big thick Ewald tubes used to wash out the stomachs of patients whose stomach outlets were obstructed from ulcer scars. Tubes were passed morning and evening, day and night.

One morning, up early as usual to do my scut work and pass my tubes, I had had ten tubes to handle, an unusually high number. As I passed the nurses' station for rounds, the chief resident said to me, "Oh Green, pass a tube on Mr. Jones and get another check on his stomach acid."

Exhausted and without thinking, I blew up. "I've passed ten tubes already this morning, and I'm damned if I'm going to pass a Levin." Everyone but me erupted in laughter at the unintended pun I had made on "eleven."

Nursing anecdotes

One of the senior surgeons insisted that all his patients receiving intravenous fluids also receive vitamins in the infusion. Believe it or not, in those days the IV bottles were open at the top, with little paper caps on them which were easily removed to add more fluid, medications, blood, whatever, in a most non-sterile fashion. The vitamin B and C mixture we used was named Berocca C; it colored the clear glucose/saline infusions yellow, so one could easily see if the vitamin had been added. One morning, while waiting for the surgeon so rounds could begin, the senior resident looked down the ward at the twenty or so beds all in a row and saw an IV in which the intravenous fluid was colorless. "Get an ampule of Berocca C into that IV," he barked at one of the residents who, in turn, barked the order at me, the intern. Not to be outdone, I repeated the order to the head nurse, and she, in turn, did so to a student nurse who had just joined the team. The surgeon arrived, and rounds started. When we arrived at the bedside in question we were shocked to see an *unopened* ampule of the vitamin floating around in the IV fluid!

Another anecdote about a nurse not quite accustomed to the routines on the service is worth recording. The first thing I usually did upon returning to the ward each morning, before getting started on my scut work, was to check the night nurses' notes about the patients. Occasionally the first sign of some complication, or an impending catastrophe, could be found there. If anything serious had occurred, of course, the routine was to call the intern on duty for telephone advice, although a trip to the ward was often necessary. The pecking order was strict: never were residents or Dave Orringer, the senior resident, to be disturbed by the nursing staff.

One morning, checking on a patient who had been operated upon the day before, I read the following in the notes.

— 1:25 a.m.
— Bright red blood noted on dressing. Dr. Orringer notified.
— 2:15 a.m.
— More bright red blood noted on dressing. Dr. Orringer notified. Told to look for signs of shock and, if found, to notify Dr. Green.
— 2:30 a.m.
— No signs of shock noted.

It was a novel way for the young nurse to learn the proper hierarchy.

A Prescient Note

Writing notes in the chart is a major aspect of any physician's record keeping. Sometimes, looking back, a written note will appear to have been remarkably prescient; other times, remarkably naive, ironic, or just plain wrong.

Another surgical attending I will call Harold Tarnow was considered something of an out of control wild man by the house staff. He had a reputation for overzealous aggressiveness. For example, one patient, a Puerto Rican man had a gigantic—I mean gigantic—hard mass over and attached to his right scapula. Although multiple biopsies had revealed it to be the fatty tissue of a benign lipoma, Tarnow had decided it might well be malignant due to its size and firmness and needed to be removed. He presumably had the patient's consent. The surgery turned out to be extremely complex, difficult and bloody. Finally, going full speed ahead and extending his resection, Tarnow did an actual forequarter amputation: he removed the tumor, part of the back, and the entire arm from the shoulder down. Dr. Otani, the pathologist, could only find benign elements in the specimen, nothing warranting such radical amputation, resulting in a lot of justified criticism of Tarnow.

Not long after, one of Tarnow's patients was admitted to my ward. A little sad and drooping lady, Mrs. Ellenberg's thyroid gland was replaced by a dense mass, which was to be removed. Strangely, no tests of her thyroid function had been done. As she gave me her history in her gravelly voice, I also noticed that her face was deeply lined and emotionless, with thickened skin. And in her chart I found a laboratory report of an elevated serum cholesterol. At surgery the mass and the entire thyroid gland were inextricably bound together, and Tarnow removed it all. Upon pathologic examination, the mass turned out to be a struma, a benign inflammatory condition of the gland.

I wrote a note in the chart: "Facies, skin and cholesterol suggested myxedema (the condition of advanced low thyroid function) preoperatively." I added that surely this condition would supervene now that the whole thyroid had been removed. Tarnow remonstrated, saying that Mrs. Ellenberg had had little or no viable thyroid to begin with, so removing the gland should make no difference. Turnow turned out to be wrong. Mrs. Ellenberg returned, some months later, in serious straits, with the lowest basal metabolic rate on record at the hospital. My ignored yet prescient note may well have reflected the lesson I had learned, in part, from Percy Klingenstein: to trust my instinct and judgment even when it differed from my superiors.

The Pathologist

Bull

Thomas Stonebrink, called "Bull" by the nurses and house staff due to his massive size, was in one of the first waves of soldiers to go ashore on D-Day, June 6, 1944, in Normandy. He had been wounded there, his spine shattered by a bullet. He was then rescued and eventually returned to the US and to the Veterans Hospital. Today specialized spinal cord injury centers offer men like him exemplary care; such was not true then. He was now a paraplegic, paralyzed from the waist down. Over the next five years Bull, a giant of a man weighing well over 200 pounds, had had many infections, primarily of the urinary tract; his buttocks and legs had suffered non-healing decubitus ulcers—pressure sores. He finally succumbed to a febrile illness, some type of a fatal infection.

Bull was my very first autopsy. The autopsy was not easy for me, because of his size and my inexperience, and because, although I had seen many autopsies, this was the first time it was I who was incising the flesh and exposing the organs of a recently living, breathing human being. I was able to determine, however, that the terminal event had been infection of one of his heart valves, the organisms probably arising from one of his skin ulcers. It was a sobering experience for me; a reminder that, although five years had passed, the war was not over, in a very real sense, for many men. It was a fitting introduction to the Veterans Administration.

After having finished my internship, I had signed on for a year of residency in Pathology at the Veterans Administration Hospital in The Bronx. (Mt. Sinai was not permitting interns interested in Internal

41

Medicine to continue immediately in their residencies—too many men, returning from World War II service and interested in further training, were on a waiting list.) I had enjoyed Pathology very much in medical school; furthermore, Pathology was considered good background for a career as a diagnostician—what many general internists were before the days of more specialization within the discipline—a position to which I then aspired.

Witnessing the "Impossible"

Something had gone terribly wrong. I could tell by the look on Jerry Sharfman's face, when I arrived one morning at the hospital. He had been awaiting my arrival. The night before, he had admitted Sven Andersson around 11 p.m. Andersson had recently developed increasing anginal chest pain. After a thorough examination and viewing an unchanged electrocardiogram, Jerry had reassured Andersson he would be fine, prescribed the usual cardiac medications, and then went to bed. A nurse awoke him at 5 a.m. to say that Andersson was unresponsive. Jerry went to his bedside and found Andersson dead; he was stunned. He noticed a giant, almost football size, swelling over his right arm, over the biceps muscle. It had not been there just hours earlier, so Jerry reasoned that, somehow, the major artery to Andersson's arm—the axillary or brachial artery—had ruptured, hemorrhaged, and caused his immediate death from shock. Sharfman pressed me to begin the autopsy and confirm his suspicion of such a rare and unusual event.

When autopsy permission is granted, unless special consent is specifically obtained, the examination is limited to the thorax and abdomen. Examining the brain, for example, requires specific authorization. In this case, Sharfman had taken care to obtain permission to examine the extremities. At his urging, in contrast to the standard procedure, I agreed to check the arm first. I did, and found a giant mass—a fatty tumor—that had to have been there for years, and without any recent bleeding. Sharfman was nonplussed. "But it wasn't there last night," he insisted.

I understood his confusion, and as gently as possible told him, "But look at it, it must have been."

He shook his head in astonishment. "It's just impossible."

Somehow, in the press of a nighttime admission, in spite of a careful exam, in spite of taking Andersson's pulse and blood pressure (obviously on the left side), Jerry had totally missed the giant lipoma. Sharfman, a medical resident whom I knew to be an excellent and careful physician, remained baffled: "I must have missed it; but I couldn't have missed it; how could I have missed it? How could I not have seen a mass of that size? It must have been there, but it couldn't have been there!"

Further examination of the body revealed widespread arteriosclerosis—hardening of the artery walls—and the pipestem coronary arteries were full of calcium and obstructed in more than one segment. Exact cause of death: heart attack.

Poor Sharfman. I bet he never failed to carefully check both arms again. And when I returned to clinical practice, neither did I, or at least I hope so. That night I witnessed just how possible it is to miss an obvious finding, no matter how impossible it seems.

The Final Arbiter

Harold Cohen, a middle-aged, markedly obese man, entered the hospital with many complaints, prominent among which were fatigue, lethargy and shortness of breath. Other than a ruddy complexion and some foot swelling, however, his physical examination had been unremarkable, his heart and lungs described as normal. His laboratory studies revealed a markedly elevated hemoglobin and red blood cell count. The other components of his blood count, the white blood cells and the platelets, were at the upper limits of normal. An excess of red blood cells indicated, in broad terms, one of two conditions. By far the most frequent, usually termed erythrocytosis (excess red blood cells) often showed up as a secondary condition, most commonly resulting from a complication of heart or lung disease. Decreased oxygen in the blood would stimulate the body to increase the number of red cells in an attempt to maintain oxygen supply to the tissues.

43

The other, less common condition was a true excess of red cells—called polycythemia rubra vera—indicating a tumor of the blood forming system. If this were the case, the blood oxygen level should be normal. The distinction between these two conditions was obviously important, as both prognosis and treatment depended upon it. (An aside: the specific test for the oxygen level in the arterial blood was, at that time, fraught with difficulty, and only a few laboratories in the country, including ours, could perform it.)

To his physician's surprise, Cohen's oxygen level was reduced, indicating the first, more common, condition of erythrocytosis, which most likely had resulted from heart or lung disease—even though both organs were seemingly normal.

Cohen's heart and lungs were studied extensively, and only a few minor abnormalities were found, consistent with his age, and perhaps, with his mild smoking history. Other rare causes of a secondary polycythemia were excluded. So how to account for his low blood oxygen, confirmed many times? One postulation was that the red blood cells themselves, having increased in mass, had somehow led to the low oxygen concentration, perhaps by their sluggish flow through the lungs. This was a hitherto undescribed phenomenon.

Cohen was treated with both oxygen supplementation and judicious removal of blood by bleeding—standard treatment, then and now—with little overall change in his condition. Eventually, further complications ensued, and Harold Cohen succumbed. Permission for the autopsy was obtained. Since his condition had been unexplained, the autopsy room was crowded with concerned and interested staff.

I proceeded eagerly, pleased to be the one to finally provide answers to Harold Cohen's perplexing case. But what I discovered not only did not reveal any answers, it actually created more questions: Harold's heart and lungs were absolutely normal. I cut here, I snipped there, but still could find nothing abnormal. Even later, when examining multiple microscopic slides with my attendings, the gross findings were confirmed: normal heart and lungs.

The clinicians were excited; something unusual was going on here. They put Mr. Cohen's case together with some others and published a major study, entitled "Pulmonary function studies in Polycythemia Vera," a report which created some controversy. And there matters stood until about ten years later. In the same medical journal, a group of physicians published another paper discussing patients who had what they called the "Pickwickian syndrome." (In Charles Dickens's novel *The Pickwick Papers*, a character named Fat Joe drops off to sleep at inappropriate times.) These patients, often obese, had some sort of sleep abnormality which led to the same behavior. Their abnormal sleep pattern was associated with absent, or inadequate, obstructed breathing, creating a lack of oxygen in the air sacs of the lungs. This, in turn, resulted in insufficient oxygen in the blood, which eventually led to heart failure— and erythrocytosis. Today the condition is commonly referred to as sleep apnea. Such a diagnosis would in retrospect explain Cohen's situation.

The road to the pursuit of truth in science is tortuous. Many apparent cul de sacs, even dead ends, may turn out to have been only curves along the way, as new findings dispel old hypotheses that seemed, at one time, to be facts. Even the autopsy, usually the final arbiter, turned out not to be so in Harold Cohen's case.

The Undertaker

It was just a few years after the war. Everybody knew the movie "Miracle on Thirty Fourth Street," and everybody knew Edmund Gwenn, the kindly Santa Claus figure. The undertaker looked just like him— short, face deeply lined with smiley furrows, blue eyes which appeared to twinkle. A man of good humor.

Just as my duty as a resident was to open up and examine the bodies, the undertaker's job was to close them back up. One bright summer Saturday morning, I autopsied a man who had suffered from extensive tuberculosis. The disease had destroyed his left lung, and left a large volume of pus in the space surrounding the lung, pus which was, undoubtedly, highly infectious. This was, by far, the worst, most extensive case of an infectious illness I had yet seen in my young career. Masked, gloved and gowned, I completed the autopsy with great care to protect myself from exposure. After I had collected all the specimens I needed for microscopic study, I went to the dressing room, changed my clothes, washed thoroughly, joked with our diener, Ralph, who kept our morgue spick and span, then returned through the autopsy room on my way home. I stopped dead in my tracks: the Edmund Gwenn undertaker was sewing up the corpse with bare, ungloved hands! A mere needle stick could quickly result in the inoculation of TB germs directly into his skin—a circumstance so frequent it had a name: prosector's wart. I had to warn him.

"Gee," I said, careful not to startle him, "that man is really *very* infectious. With TB. I would strongly advise you to put on gloves."

"Doc, I know," he said, "but I really can't do a good job sewing him up with gloves on. I need to have the proper feeling in my hands."

"Well," I returned, "I understand, but this case is *really* extreme." Silence. "I think you ought to be wearing gloves anyway."

"Thanks, Doc," he said in a tone implying that young whippersnapper doctors didn't understand the real world. He went back to work, ignoring my advice. I understood that the artist in him took precedence over the practical man; nevertheless, I thought him foolish.

Much later that year, on a gloomy winter Saturday, I again performed an autopsy on a tuberculous patient. The body was that of a young black man, wasted away to almost nothing, except for an abdomen swollen full of cheesy tuberculous material from tuberculosis of the peritoneal cavity, its lymph nodes, and indeed, all the abdominal structures, resulting in an unusual giant mass of destroyed infected tissue—even more extensive than the earlier case. Once more, after completing my work under carefully protected conditions, I returned to the morgue. I found my cheery undertaker at work but, with pleasant surprise, I noticed that this time he was wearing gloves.

"Oh, good for you," I said. "I'm glad to see you realized how contagious he is."

"Oh, it's not that, Doc," he said. "He's a nigger, and I can't bear to touch their skin." *Their* skin, not his. And he smiled.

I never again thought of the undertaker as the kindly Santa Claus figure.

Look All Over

During the remainder of my residency in Internal Medicine, I visited the autopsy room on occasion, when one of my patients, or one I knew, died. I would also check their microscopic slides; but otherwise, my contact with Pathology was limited.

My residency neared its completion, and the government informed me that I owed them eighteen months of service in return for supporting me during World War II. I joined the Public Health Service to meet this obligation, after having arranged for an appointment in the Indian Bureau which, at that time, was under the supervision of the Interior Department. Tuberculosis was a common ailment among Native Americans, and my interest in the Indian Bureau stemmed from my desire to practice chest disease. I liked the idea of providing good care and service to a segment of the population that was greatly in need of competent medical care; it appealed to my sense of social justice. After a short stay in Albuquerque, New Mexico working as an assistant at the Indian Bureau Tuberculosis Sanatorium, I was offered, and accepted, the position of Chief of the Tuberculosis division of 160 beds at the Talihina Medical Center, an Indian Bureau hospital in Talihina, Oklahoma. The opportunity to run a sanatorium of 160 beds, always full of patients, greatly appealed to me.

It was also a fascinating time to work in tuberculosis. New medications were coming on board to replace the days when bed rest and collapse therapy (a procedure in which the infected lung is immobilized in an effort to allow it to rest and recover) were the basic treatments for tuberculous patients. I felt I might be able to offer patients more modern, more sophisticated medicine, and I relished the opportunity.

I was one of only three physicians on staff when I arrived in early 1952. Shortly after my arrival one of my patients died, not an unusual occurrence in those days. Aspects of her illness had been confusing. After the body was removed to the funeral home in town I spoke to the undertaker: could I perform an autopsy there? Yes, indeed. He was pleased to have the opportunity to witness a dissection. The undertaker's name was David Drake; over the next three years he and I and our families became great friends.

Nicholas Romine was an elderly Choctaw man who lived with his family in an isolated cabin in adjacent Pushmataha county. His sons brought him to our hospital after he had lost a large quantity of blood from his mouth. One might think it simple to tell whether such a hemorrhage is due to coughing or vomiting, but in reality it is often not. Patients who vomit blood often aspirate some of it into their lungs and cough; patients who are bleeding from the lungs often swallow much of the blood and then vomit it up. This was true with Nicholas, and the family said such hemorrhaging had happened before. The prior spring he had suddenly experienced a massive gushing of blood from his mouth. They took him to Antlers, a nearby city, where he saw a physician who hospitalized him. As a massive hemorrhage is much more common from the gastrointestinal tract than from the lungs, a GI series—a study in which the patient swallows barium for x-rays of the stomach and duodenum—had been done. The physician had told the family that Romine probably had a bleeding ulcer. Fortunately, Romine's hemorrhage had ceased, and he had returned home. Now the hemorrhage had recurred, so the family brought him to Talihina.

Although his blood count was low, Nicholas was not in shock and did not require transfusion. He was in excellent general condition for a man almost 90. I was not certain if this was hemoptysis—coughed up bleeding from the lungs, or hematemesis—vomited bleeding from the stomach, but in any case I promptly took a chest x-ray. I was not surprised when it was abnormal, but it did not reveal the characteristic tuberculosis that I had half expected, and which was so common among my patients. Instead I saw a large orange-sized density in the middle lobe of Romine's right lung. I was certain I had found the source of the bleeding.

Bleeding from the lungs is frightening for patients. Since it was a problem I faced often with my tuberculous patients, I had developed a step by step program in which I tried multiple remedies to control the bleeding. Although I had little evidence of success with any one remedy, going through each step served, at the very least, to reduce anxiety for my patients, the nurses and, I must admit, me. I put Romine on this program, even though his condition differed from my TB patients.

48

Meanwhile, I still had no clear diagnosis for Romine. Faced with an uncommon finding, I knew that unusual manifestations of common diseases are always more likely than uncommon diseases, so tuberculosis was still a possibility; perhaps he had an unusual manifestation of it. But the tests for TB were negative. The x-ray shadow was surely compatible with lung cancer. However, despite the fact that my Indian patients were often heavy smokers, this condition was surprisingly uncommon among them. In addition, at that time, studies had suggested that the middle lobe was an uncommon site for lung cancer. Another condition, termed "the right middle lobe syndrome," seemed a more likely possibility. In this situation a compromised bronchus—the airway which led to the rest of the lobe—causes multiple infections within this particular lobe.

I treated Romine with a course of antibiotics, even though he had few signs of infection. One of the major steps in my program was using Ceanothyn, a liquid mixture of multiple ingredients dissolved in a generous volume of alcohol, much more than in the ordinary tincture. I had come across it shortly after my arrival at the hospital. It was one among dozens of ancient herbal remedies (most of which I had never heard of) down in a large storage room in the hospital's basement. Romine loved the Ceanothyn, and ascribed his improvement to it—and I was unwilling to disabuse him of his confidence. Indeed, his hemorrhage gradually subsided. The density in the lung also shrunk somewhat, but the bulk of it remained. Whether his improvement was spontaneous or due to my treatment, I did not know.

As he recovered, we faced the question of how to proceed. I had no additional methods of testing, such as special x-rays or bronchoscopy, available to me. Romine could go to a major hospital in Oklahoma City or Tulsa for further study, but the family was clearly reluctant to travel, given his advanced age. Romine and his family only wished to return home. I did not consider more prolonged antibiotic therapy, which would have been a novel approach at the time.

I then did two things that I still wonder about, medically and ethically, when I think back. First, I supplied the family with a dozen or so bottles of Ceanothyn for him to use as needed. I told them, of course, that the hemorrhage might recur and might be fatal, if more massive.

49

As for the second, I said an autopsy would reveal to all of us what his terminal condition had been, if Romine died. They agreed and signed an undated autopsy permission before they left.

Three months later Romine's son appeared. Dad was doing fine, but he had run out of Ceanothyn. Might they have some more? I gave him the remaining half dozen bottles from the basement shelves and wished them well.

Later that year I got a phone call from the undertaker of a funeral home in Antlers: Romine had bled again and died. I arrived later that day and prepared to do the autopsy. I also called the physician, whom I will call Dr. Butler, who had treated Romine for his initial episode and invited him to be present at the autopsy. To my surprise and pleasure, he immediately came to the funeral home. He was a well-trained osteopathic physician from Michigan, who appreciated the opportunity to witness the autopsy and discuss Romine's case.

Butler was somewhat dismayed when I demonstrated that Romine's stomach and duodenum were entirely normal, without evidence of an ulcer or scarring from a prior one, as Butler had previously thought. The right middle lobe was shrunken and entirely hollowed out, representing the remains of a destroyed infected lobe with no signs of either tuberculosis or cancer. So my diagnosis had been correct, though my being right had not particularly helped the old man.

After the autopsy, Butler invited me back to his office to visit and to talk medicine. While there, he pulled Romine's x-rays from his files. The stomach and duodenum did not look abnormal to me. At the top of these abdominal x-rays, one could also clearly see the bottom of the chest and lower portions of the lungs. And there it was: the abnormal shadow in the right middle lobe, smaller than when he had seen me. Butler was abashed. If he had recognized the abnormality on Romine's first visit, it was possible, although unlikely, that antibiotic therapy might have led to a better outcome. It was an important lesson of remembering to look at *all* of the film, not only at the organs specifically under study.

It would not be the last time the principle of Look All Over, be it for physical examination or x-rays, would be confirmed.

The Trial

Zeke Face was considered sort of a sad sack in Talihina. He had contracted polio as a child, which left him with a bad left leg and visible limp. His physical defect, no doubt, contributed to his personality: shy and insecure. He could be seen doing odd jobs around town. One thing in Zeke's favor was his marriage to Alice, a pretty woman, although questions had been raised about her fidelity.

Dick Oakland was a big bluff guy, a contractor from McAlester, the nearest city of even moderate size to Talihina. He had been in town for some time on a construction project. The rumors abounded concerning Oakland and Alice.

One night my friend, David Drake, the undertaker, was called by the police to come to Zeke and Alice's house—Dick Oakland had been shot and killed. Zeke Face was arrested on the spot for murder. The story was that Zeke had come home, found Oakland there with his wife, and shot him. At the funeral home one of the investigating policemen remarked that it was a shame no coroner was around these parts, so that the bullets could be recovered. David told them about me, and that surely I could get the bullets out. I was called in by the police, I think somewhat reluctantly, and asked to retrieve the bullets as quickly as possible.

I performed the autopsy at David's funeral home, as always, but this time with the police all standing around watching. I found two bullet entry wounds, both not from very close range. One was in the upper left arm, just below the shoulder; the other was in the upper left front of the chest. Rather than a formal autopsy, I decided to follow the bullet openings and tracks.

The first bullet was easy to find. The track showed it had entered the arm, traversed under the skin towards the midline, hit the breastbone, fractured it and then bounced off. The bullet lay in the nearby tissues. Clearly it was not the fatal shot.

The second bullet gave me a problem. The track went directly into the front of the left lung, where I found a lot of blood in the pleural cavity, the space between the lung and the ribs. The track in the lung went mostly downwards, slightly backwards and to the right, exiting the lung at its medial edge, then entering the heart. The pericardial space around the heart contained some blood, but the track went gradually backwards right through the heart, straight down the interventricular septum which separates the two ventricles. The damage was obviously fatal, but I could find no bullet! I was now working deep within the body, without very good exposure, and the police were getting impatient.

The bullet had exited the heart to the right, and I finally found it, deep in the tissues of the abdomen, behind the liver. Now with the gun and two bullets in hand, the cops left to do ballistic studies.

A few months later I, along with David and several Talihina residents, was notified and asked to be present as an expert witness at the trial. John Murphy, the prosecuting attorney—a young man said to have political ambition—interviewed me briefly prior to the trial, asking about my findings. The trial itself took place in Poteau, the county seat of Leflore County, and many Talihina residents attended—a murder was big news.

During the trial, witnesses were not allowed in the court room for the early parts of the trial. My very clear memory is of waiting in a side room—not unlike a Hollywood movie—and playing their version of euchre—high low jack and game. Lots of laughter, whooping, southern accents, cowboy hats, boots and denim, smoking, and card slapping occurred around that table. It was hard to believe I was an actual participant in what felt like a very surreal situation.

Finally, I was called into the courtroom to testify as a prosecution witness. The scene, once more, reminded me of that in a movie: a warm day in a sunlit wooden courtroom, jurors wearing mostly dungarees and boots, a non-robed judge sporting a bolo tie, lots of spectators fanning themselves. I was sworn in and asked about my credentials. I gave them. I was then questioned about the bullet removal. I explained how I had retrieved them. The district attorney ended his questioning there. The defense had no questions. I was excused.

I was amazed I hadn't been asked my opinion of what actually occurred based on the evidence. Everybody knew the story the defense offered: Zeke Face had come home and found Oakland there. They had had words. Oakland, who was much bigger, had then come at Zeke as if to attack him. Zeke had pulled out his gun in self defense and fired two shots. Oakland fell, dead. That was it.

But the bullet tracks told a different story.

One bullet had been fired when Oakland's side was facing Zeke, going straight through as it did. That could happen if they were both standing, but not facing each other, or if Oakland had been lying on the floor, right side down. But if this were the case, the bullet entry would show the shot being fired from closer range. And if Oakland was on the floor, then the second shot would have had to have been fired at a crazy, rather unlikely, angle, to enter the front of the left chest and travel as it did. I thought about it, and thought about it, drawing many theoretical pictures of the body with various shot angles. I could come up with only one conclusion: Zeke Face was lying about Oakland coming at him. The evidence strongly indicated that the first shot was the one in the arm, fired with both men standing, Oakland's side facing towards Zeke. Oakland then started to turn and to fall, and the second shot entered his left front chest going backwards, down and to the right—the course my autopsy had shown it had taken—as he did so. It was the only logical explanation. Admittedly, I was not trained as a forensic pathologist. But I felt confident in my opinion that Zeke's story of Oakland coming at him was patently untrue.

The jury was unable to reach a verdict—a hung jury, said to be mostly for acquittal. Why? And why had I not been asked about the inferences from the bullet track direction, which should have been major evidence for the prosecution? Zeke Face was never re-tried.

David explained it to me. The story around town was that when Zeke Face had come home, he and Oakland had had words. Alice had been silent. Face questioned Oakland, who dismissed him as irrelevant, a nobody, a weakling, not much of a man. Face shot him. But in spite of Face having committed the crime, the region's sympathy was with him, not Oakland. This wasn't because Zeke was the local, and Oakland, the outsider, nor because Zeke had a crippled leg, nor even because of his wife's presumed infidelity, but because, as David Drake succinctly put it, "Bob, Dick Oakland sassed him in his own home."

I didn't press David, but it was clear to me that in his mind, and in the minds of our Oklahoma "western" residents, you just didn't sass a man in his own home. No matter what the circumstances. In their minds, the killing was justified.

I Sigh

Myra Ray Dies

Funeral services were held at Good Creek church, near Clayton, for Myra Ruth Ray, teenage daughter of Mr.and Mrs. Eber Ray, of Talihina. Rev. R. A. Walker conducted the services. Burial was in the Good Creek cemetery, under the direction of the Drake Funeral Home.

Myra Ruth was born November 15, 1937 in Idabel. She died on February 4 after a month's illness. She is survived by her parents and her brother and sister: Bobby Joe and Paula Jane. Myra Ruth was a member of the Talihina Baptist Church.

Talihina American, February 9, 1954

Myra was 16, in high school. Her records showed multiple clinic visits to our hospital since she had been a baby, but basically she was a healthy young Choctaw girl. That is, until she suddenly came down with a high fever, shaking chills, cough and shortness of breath. Doc Johnson in town diagnosed "double pneumonia"; she was promptly hospitalized under my care. I found a confused and very sick young lady: her temperature was over 103, her pulse rate 140, and her respirations unusually rapid at 40 breaths per minute. She had multiple herpetic blisters—cold sores—around her mouth, often seen with pneumonia. Her chest exam showed fairly typical findings of lobar pneumonia in the left lower lobe of her lung, which was confirmed by a chest x-ray. Her white blood cell count was markedly elevated, and she was mildly anemic. I aspirated some secretions from her throat; a stain revealed many pus cells, but fewer organisms than I had expected, although those present were compatible with a diagnosis of pneumonia. Since our lab facilities were limited, I could not culture her blood.

I agreed with the diagnosis of severe lobar pneumonia, and although she was very, very ill, I assumed the massive doses of penicillin I administered would turn her illness around. I reassured her father, who worked at the hospital. Over the next few days, however, she showed no improvement; in fact, her condition worsened. Myra became more anemic and was frequently delirious. We provided oxygen by tent in those days; she would refuse to remain in the tent. Her breathing became so rapid that she had difficulty swallowing even fluids. I began to worry. I switched her treatment to a broad spectrum antibiotic. A week had passed with no apparent response.

That evening my wife and I were visiting with our friends, the Drakes. At one point David asked, "How's Myra Ruth doin'? Is her pneumonia gettin' any better?" We had been in Talihina almost two years, and I had become accustomed to the local attitudes, as they related to the concept of privacy. Here, there were few secrets, if any; everyone, and not maliciously, seemed to know everyone else's business. So instead of being shocked or offended by David's question, I simply replied that she was not doing well.

"I'm not surprised," said David, "I figured it probably was TB anyway."

I was surprised and alarmed. "David, what do you mean?"

"Well," he said, "everybody knows Etta (Myra's mother) has had TB for years and has refused treatment. That poor girl Myra Ruth is the one who takes care of her and the whole family." I was shocked. Myra's failure to respond could be due to an overwhelming acute tuberculous pneumonia, a rare, but not unheard of, manifestation of TB!

The next morning I spoke to Myra's father, who confirmed David's story. I insisted Etta be brought in and, sure enough, her x-ray showed advanced TB in both lungs, her sputum heavily positive. I examined Myra's sputum, but found no TB germs. Nevertheless, I felt certain of my course, and I immediately began anti-tuberculosis treatment with my two mainstay medicines: isoniazid, which would only affect the TB germ, and streptomycin, which could be active against other organisms as well.

To my distress, Myra still showed no improvement. Her delirium and her irrationality worsened; she became incontinent and semi-comatose at times. Her anemia progressed, requiring transfusion. She had now been under my care for two weeks, with no change for the better. I examined her spinal fluid; it was normal. I considered a radical intervention: cortisone. As the first adrenal steroid in clinical use, it had become available only a few years earlier. Cortisone had proved successful against some overwhelming infections, as long as the infection itself was known, and the patient was "covered" by the appropriate antibiotic. This was not the situation with Myra—as I had no specific bacteriologic diagnosis, I certainly wasn't prescribing the "appropriate" antibiotic—but I was desperate. With great trepidation I began cortisone in moderate doses, even for that time, and continued it for two days. To my great disappointment there was no apparent change in Myra. I stopped the steroid treatment.

Then over the next few days Myra seemed to be improving: her fever came down a bit, and she was able to swallow some fluid. But again, she relapsed. She began to bleed into her skin, vomiting blood and showing evidence of blood in her stool. Eventually Myra's temperature spiked to 105, and her vital signs deteriorated. Near the end of the fourth week, she died.

I performed the autopsy upon Myra's remains, undoubtedly the most difficult one emotionally I have ever done. The findings were surprisingly unremarkable: I found fresh "consolidation" suggesting pneumonia in the right lung, and more chronic changes in the left lower lobe. It did not really look tuberculous, but I convinced myself that TB was possible. Her other organs were grossly unremarkable. I sent specimens for microscopic examination not only to Bethesda, but also to my old pathology consultant in The Bronx. Their reports were similar—there was no tuberculosis; the lungs showed acute and chronic organizing pneumonia. The adrenal glands were depleted of fat, suggesting an eventual inadequate response to the stress of the illness. The Bethesda pathologist concluded: "these findings point to an overwhelming infection as the cause of death."

Even today lobar pneumonia—due to the commonest organism that causes it, "the pneumococcus"—is not uniformly cured. Fatalities occur more often in the elderly, those with compromised immune systems, and following influenza. Death is less common in young, presumably healthy, people, but it occurs. I believe in Myra's case the germs had probably invaded her blood stream, causing sepsis or septicemia, or in layman's terms, blood poisoning. Her illness may also have been complicated by

DIC (disseminated intravascular coagulation), a condition which had not yet been described. In any case, now in hindsight, I can see that the possibility of tuberculosis was clearly a red herring; it may have kept me from more aggressive general antibiotic chemotherapy. I believe my decision to try steroids, cortisone, was correct; but I regret not using larger doses and continuing them for longer. Of all my patients for whom my care has been inadequate, I feel the worst about Myra Ruth.

Even now, as I write, I sigh and sigh again for the life I did not save.

In the vast majority of cases, the autopsy remains the final arbiter, often settling conflicting opinions and findings, when performed. Autopsies were still done quite frequently in the post World War II years. The immediate cause of death, as well as the background cause of the patient's fatal illness, was often unknown at the time of death. In fact, the autopsy rate—the percentage of deaths in which autopsies were performed at any given hospital—was considered a measure of quality, was reported to and by reviewing bodies, and looked at carefully by physicians applying for medical training. That is no longer true; advances in technique, particularly in imaging studies, now establish diagnoses most of the time during life, and—unfortunately—the autopsy is less common than it once was, although when done often continues to surprise.

I had enjoyed Pathology in Medical School, and I chose it for my post-internship year. I never regretted the decision and found the experience immensely helpful in preparation for the next step in my medical education—the VA Hospital in The Bronx.

In The Bronx

It Was So Obvious

It was a very hot summer day during the second year of my residency at the Veterans Administration Hospital in The Bronx. After my year in Pathology, I had decided to stay on at the VA Hospital in Internal Medicine. The VA was an old facility and very definitely not air conditioned. I had been told a new admission was on his way to the ward and, sweltering, I awaited him.

Luigi Martini presented a bizarre sight when he limped into my examining room. Tall and skinny, he was continually mopping his sweating forehead with a soiled handkerchief. He was jumpy, twitchy, all his muscles seemingly in action. Was he staring at me? It was hard to tell—one eye didn't seem to move; the other seemed to stare, but then darted here and there.

I introduced myself, then began with my usual opening, why had he come to the hospital? Luigi, mopping away, said, "10% service connected for gastritis."

"What?!" I could barely conceal my amazement, having expected him to report a symptom: pain, fever, weight loss, whatever.

Again he repeated, "10% service connected for gastritis." Fortunately, he carried his referral from the Regional Office of the Veterans Administration with him.

"Hold on a minute," I said, "let me check your records."

And what a story they told! In the waning days of World War II, Martini had literally been blown up and almost apart by a land mine. Immediate treatment had saved his life; eventually transferred to Walter Reed Medical Center, he had been hospitalized for almost four—*four!*—years, and had undergone *twenty-three* major surgical procedures. He had a plate in his skull, a glass eye, full dentures, damaged ear drums and hearing, a partially paralyzed left arm, and an artificial below-the-knee right leg prosthesis. Remarkably, after the four years, he had married one of his nurses and had been discharged to civilian life. He subsequently developed indigestion and had lost weight; a diagnosis of gastritis, inflammation of the stomach, had been made previously during one of his multiple abdominal procedures. The Army rated Martini as 100% disabled; 10% of that calculation related to the gastritis, which accounted for his bizarre presenting complaint. He had been referred to the hospital for further evaluation of that condition.

I examined Luigi. He was a mass of scar tissue, literally from head to toe. His abdomen, tender all over, was criss-crossed with evidence of his wounds and surgical scars. While I did my examination, we talked. He was having some difficulty adjusting to civilian life. He didn't know what to do, what his future would hold. He was jumpy, and he sweated profusely. Although his muscles were normal, his reflexes were very active. Other than his thinness, a rapid pulse and his obvious nervousness, his exam was normal—a peculiar phrase to use for a man so covered with scars.

The diagnosis was pretty obvious to me. I would institute the proper studies, as requested, for his stomach condition, but it was clear what was wrong with this poor fellow. After four years of a sheltered existence, he now had a new wife and had to face the stresses of independent civilian life. Understandably, it was simply too much for him. Frailty, and nerves, thy name is Martini. I awaited an interview with his wife, planning to suggest some counseling or psychiatric help.

The next morning as was routine, my attending physician arrived to go on rounds with me and to evaluate my new patient. Although I respected him, I did not get along well with this particular man. He was a professor at Columbia-Presbyterian, obviously competent and experienced, but he was always too serious and inflexible, over-attentive to irrelevant detail, with no sense of humor. On this hot summer day, he wore a heavy gray flannel suit with a vest, shirt and tie. He spoke to Luigi and examined him. He noticed the sweating and the fast pulse. He had Luigi follow his moving finger with his one good eye. He said, "I think his lid lags a bit as he moves his eye down. You had better check him out for Graves' disease."

Graves' disease is a term for serious overactivity of the thyroid gland. We had always been taught that it was a good idea to exclude organic illness prior to making a psychiatric diagnosis, but it seemed to me in this instance that my attending's suggestion was just silly. The basis for Martini's illness was so obvious! Nevertheless, I complied with the attending's suggestion. The usual test to check thyroid function at that time was the BMR, or basal metabolic rate. However, it required intact ear drums, which Luigi did not have. Fortunately, a new test, the radioactive iodine uptake, was available. The thyroid gland has an extreme avidity for iodine; when a small amount of radioactive iodine is administered, it is "taken up," that is, concentrated by the gland, and thus the function of the thyroid can be evaluated.

A couple of days later my friend Sol Berson, then head of our radioisotope division, came rushing up to the ward to see Martini. (Berson later was the inventor of a process called radio-immunoassay, a major medical research procedure; after his death his colleague, Rosalyn Yalow, won the Nobel prize.) Despite the fact that Luigi's thyroid gland was barely palpable by any of us, his uptake was the highest ever seen in our laboratory or of which Berson was aware! Chalk up one for my attending physician. (We later learned that a stressful life event is a trigger for Graves' disease.)

The treatment was simple: a large dose of radioactive iodine. The radiation destroyed most of the gland and restored it to normal functioning. Martini was discharged.

That fall, I saw Luigi for a follow-up, three months after his initial visit. He was no longer mopping his brow, and it wasn't only because the weather had turned cooler. He had gained thirty pounds, which put him in his normal weight range. No longer anxious, he sat in his chair comfortably, placidly, his pretty wife at his side. They had invested in a small grocery store. Oh yes, she said, this is the Luigi I met and married; it surely wasn't the Luigi I had met and mis-diagnosed! What had seemed so obvious to me was simply wrong—a terrific reminder of the precept, "Things are not always what they seem."

Triumph!

Morris Singer hobbled slowly and painfully onto the ward late one afternoon. His story was simple. He worked on a farm in New Jersey, and a week or so before, while cleaning out the stable, he had stepped on a broken, rusty nail, which pierced his heel. A more classic case of a tetanus risk can hardly be found. It was recognized as such, and tetanus antiserum was the treatment of choice to prevent the dreaded onset of tetanus itself. He was tested for a reaction to it, had none, and the prescribed dose was administered. Nevertheless, the day before admission to my ward, Morris developed fever, a rash, a general ill feeling, and painful joints, particularly in his ankles, which were swollen and tender. This collection of symptoms was also classic, evidence of a reaction to the treatment known as serum sickness.

The diagnosis was clear, but what about treatment? Pain relief, compresses to his feet, and a recently discovered antihistamine offered the possibility of slow improvement. Then I had a bright idea. Cortisone. It was the first of the adrenal steroid drugs so commonly used in medical practice today; it had then been proven effective for certain forms of arthritis. More important, it was understood that the drug worked by interfering with reactions between certain usually foreign substances (antigens) and reactants formed within the body (antibodies) to combat allergy to them. I had not read of any such use, but it seemed to me that if the mechanism of proposed action was correct, serum sickness would be an ideal condition for which cortisone should at least be helpful, if not curative.

One problem: our hospital had not yet added cortisone to its formulary, so we had none on hand for prescription. The only cortisone available was being used in a research study for treatment of patients with Hodgkin's disease. Little vials of oily, injectable cortisone, each labeled by patient, were refrigerated on the ward. But—I knew that some of the patients in the study had died. I checked the refrigerator. Sure enough, I found three vials labeled for deceased patients, each containing a small amount of residual cortisone. I drew up each remnant into a syringe, resulting in what was then a hefty dose (though today it would be considered minimal). I neither asked Singer for his consent, nor told him what I was doing, nor that what I was doing was, in a clear sense, experimental. I just injected the material into his buttock. Note, the physician-patient relationship has since changed.

The next morning I was greeted by Singer, who was waiting for me at my office door, smiling, even laughing, literally dancing, loose, supple, and pain free. Triumph! I discharged him later that day. The fact that the cortisone was in oil probably delayed its absorption, and thus prolonged its effect.

For a young house officer in training, I was proud of my creative approach; I felt smugly satisfied with my success. I did not see Singer in follow-up. I can only hope the cortisone's influence outlasted his continuing serum sickness reaction, and so justified my smugness.

An Apt Simile

Stefano Karadzmaitis complained of weakness and fatigue. A blood count revealed that he was anemic of a type that suggested blood loss, and therefore, internal bleeding. He was admitted for study and diagnosis. Steve, a short man, was still in his fifties, but he looked older. His wizened face had a perpetual grin, and his still abundant hair hung down over his eyes.

When I examined him he was indeed pale, consistent with the reported anemia. Although he said he had lost weight, he did not appear thin. My primary attention was to his abdomen; it was a bit fuller than I would have expected from the appearance of his chest and extremities. I palpated it; it was not tender or rigid. However, below his umbilicus I could feel a significant abnormality, a large mass the size of a volleyball. I recorded my finding in the chart: "arising out of the pelvis there is a large soft, yet firm, freely moveable non-tender mass, reminiscent of a pregnant uterus," which, of course, I knew wasn't the case. When my colleagues saw my written note, I was subjected to ribald mockery for my choice of words.

The gastrointestinal tract is the usual source of internal bleeding, and chemical tests on Stefano's stool were positive for occult blood. A barium enema showed a normal colon, the large intestine. However, when an upper GI series was performed, the findings were remarkable. The stomach was normal, but a while after the barium had entered the small intestine, it suddenly spread out. More and more barium was added; it seemed to collect in some sort of gigantic space, forming a straight line across the entire abdomen: barium below, air above. We were stupefied; if the material was running through a perforation in the intestine into the peritoneal cavity, we should have seen signs of peritonitis, but none were present. So what sort of structure could explain this unique finding? Our lack of answers demanded exploratory surgery.

I went to the operating room to observe Karadzmaitis's bizarre situation. The surgeon found a giant tumorous mass involving the lower portion of the small intestine. Its inner portions had hollowed out, thus establishing a direct connection and communication with the open interior of the bowel. It was into this mass that the barium had run; it was also clearly the mass I had felt on physical examination. The tumor and the adjacent bowel were removed.

Under the microscope the tumor type was a leiomyoma, not a rare form of small bowel tumor; however, this was an unusually large one. The fascinating thing is leiomyoma is exactly the same tumor type as that found in so-called fibroid tumors of the uterus. So my initial description of it feeling like a pregnant uterus had validity: the outer lining of the uterus and the mass were the same tissue. In one case the interior contained a fetus, in the other, only fluid.

Many students, residents and attending physicians had examined Karadzmaitis because of the unusual physical finding; he was a "great case." Each person properly considers himself unique; Stefano caused me to realize that to doctors, some patients are more unique than others! In any case, the outcome for Stefano Karadzmaitis, who left the hospital feeling well, was excellent. And I was pleased that my instinct to describe my initial findings as "a pregnant uterus" in a male patient had validity, despite the derision it received from colleagues.

An Age-Old Debate

In the *Archives of Internal Medicine 1999*:159:1082-87 you will find a paper entitled "Diagnosing pneumonia by physical examination: relevant or relic?" I have heard that argument ever since I have been in medicine. Today, each advance in technology, particularly in imaging, increases the concern that the physical exam is becoming more and more unnecessary and irrelevant.

In my field, lung disease, I considered myself particularly adept at the physical exam. I learned it well during my training; I honed my skills examining all my tuberculous patients in the Indian Bureau; I further sharpened them during my four years on staff at the Bronx VA. I taught the physical exam by lecture and by example. Later I wrote a section of a textbook on it. The physical exam is something I believe every physician should know how to do and know how to do well; in some situations, the physical exam is a desirable complement to modern imaging for accurate diagnosis.

In my text, I discuss the four traditional aspects of the chest exam in the sick patient: inspection, palpation, percussion and auscultation. I also added a fifth: inspection of the chest x-ray. I wasn't critical of other physicians or my trainees if an abnormal finding in the chest physical exam was missed; but if the chest x-ray, reviewed subsequently, showed an abnormality, I expected a repeat of the physical examination in order to see what the true physical findings were. I insisted the x-ray then be reexamined as well. I called this principle "Back and Forth." Its proper application should lead to a correct interpretation of findings, and most often, it does. (Although, unfortunately, many instances occur in which neither the chest x-ray nor the physical exam is sufficient for diagnosis.)

Historically, it took time and experience for a balance between the two to become routine. Tuberculosis physicians, for example, were amazingly adept at eliciting abnormal findings in the chest with only a physical exam. When x-rays started to become more common in the 1920s, radiologists were able to demonstrate very early tuberculous changes in the lungs. However, many chest men denied that x-ray abnormalities could be significant, if they could not elicit a change in the physical exam. That attitude then changed rapidly, perhaps swinging too far in the opposite direction. It is said that Merrill Sosman, a Harvard radiologist, had a stethoscope hanging in a cabinet. Under it a sign read, "a medieval instrument formerly used in the diagnosis of lung disease."

By 1948, when I was a senior in medical school, the chest x-ray was firmly established as a valuable routine exam. The physical exam, however, remained a vital part of medicine. And, in fact, at the other end of the spectrum from the Merrill Sosmans are physicians like Leroy Sloan, a distinguished community practitioner. I recall this pearl he dropped during a clinical presentation back in med school: "If you find dullness and diminished breath sounds at the lung base, stick in a needle." Those findings surely do suggest a pleural effusion, probably more common then than other abnormalities that can cause the same findings. He made no mention of any necessity for obtaining a chest x-ray to confirm his suspicions. That would be unheard of today.

All this serves to introduce Clem Hooper. In my last months of residency at the Bronx VA before I entered the Indian Bureau, I worked in the outpatient area. Clem, a vigorous healthy man in his thirties, came in complaining of chills and fever. He also had minimal symptoms of cough, sputum production and chest pain. Pneumonia was my primary concern from his history, so I examined his chest carefully. From the back, his lungs were normal, but high up anteriorly just under his right clavicle, the percussion note was dull and his breath sounds were different. Although the changes were subtle and I heard no crackles, I felt confident in my findings and marked his sheet "Admit—Pneumonia RUL." The bureaucracy, however, required that all admissions had to be approved by Dr. Samuel Goldman, Chief of Staff, who supervised the clinics. I brought the sheet to him. He read it, and said, "Where's the chest x-ray report?" I told him I hadn't ordered an x-ray, since the diagnosis was clear. Sam said, "You can't diagnose pneumonia without a chest x-ray." I knew I was a better clinician than Sam, who wasn't interested in seeing the patient. After some rather heated discussion, we compromised—he permitted the admission, and I ordered the x-ray to be taken on the way to the ward.

The next afternoon I went up to the floor to see how Clem was doing. Passing his bed, I noticed that he looked about the same. I picked up his chart only to discover that the ward physician and an attending physician had diagnosed Clem "FUO"—fever of unknown origin—based on his presentation and their own finding of a normal chest exam. Consequently, no antibiotic had been prescribed; instead, multiple tests had been ordered. I grabbed the resident, took him to the bedside, and demonstrated the exam. To my distress, I was unable to convince him of the changes. He told me he had been unable to locate the chest x-ray. Suddenly I was extremely interested in seeing it, sure that it would confirm my diagnosis. Fortunately, the x-ray showed up later that day, indicating a solid lobar pneumonia of the right upper lobe. I had been right all along. Clem then received proper treatment.

I wish I could say Clem's case was unique in my experience, but sadly it was not. The experience did, at least, help me develop confidence in my competence to perform a sophisticated chest examination.

Perhaps not surprisingly the examination debate continues among physicians: *The New England Journal of Medicine* published an article on the demise of the physical exam as recently as January, 2006—as if that were something new!

Let Your Curiosity Lead You

Diagnoses are most commonly made after relatively routine approaches—obtaining a patient's history, a set of social and system-related questions, a physical exam, and then laboratory studies, if deemed necessary after such questions and examination. A skill rarely appreciated comes from asking an unusual or creative question, which may be key to the diagnosis. I summarized this principle as "Let Your Curiosity Lead You."

Richard Moran was admitted to the Dermatology service for a gigantic basal cell cancer of the face. Most basal cells, the most common skin cancer, are diagnosed when fairly small. They can be treated by multiple methods, and are almost always curable. If left alone they do not metastasize, that is, spread to other parts of the body, but they do grow and grow locally, undermining adjacent tissues. They ulcerate, leaving a bloody surface. A lay term for them is "rodent ulcer," raising the perspective of a rat chewing away at tissue. Ugh!

Richard Moran typified an advanced case. He was a big man, six feet six inches tall, and weighing over 250 pounds. He had neglected, probably for years, what started as a pimple on his right cheek. Now the ulcer had destroyed the cheek almost to the ear, the right side of his nose, the corner of his mouth and his right lower eye lid. It was an immense tumor.

There was nothing much else in his story. He was fifty-eight years old, unmarried, a blacksmith by trade, a World War I veteran and a smoker. He gave no history of chest or lung surgery or injury; in fact, he absolutely denied any symptoms, except for those related to his face.

However, his chest x-ray, mandatory for all admissions in those days, showed a small, somewhat difficult to see shadow low in the right chest. The radiologist suggested it was a solitary pulmonary nodule, one cause of which is cancer. Given the giant tumor on the face, it was conceivable—although highly unlikely—that the cancer had spread to the lung. Laminagrams—tomograms—were obtained. This specialized x-ray procedure has now long been supplanted by CT scans—computerized tomograms—which provide excellent cross sectional views of the body.

The tomogram worked like this: the patient lay on his back on the x-ray table. By a complex system of motion of the x-ray tube and the x-ray film, back to front "slices" of the lung were created and visualized by blurring out the tissues in front and behind the slice seen most clearly. (Skeptics called them blurrograms.) A standard order was for AP (meaning anterior-posterior) tomograms 4-17 cm. Each slice was labeled by a number, for example 4 or 6, which represented the distance in centimeters measured upwards from the table.

I was consulted. My history taking from Richard Moran added nothing, and my physical examination of his chest was entirely normal. I reviewed the tomograms. Because he was such a big man, the radiologist had extended them further anteriorly than usual, all the way up to 21 cm. He had interpreted them as revealing the nodule in the middle lobe of the lung, which is a lobe in the anterior chest. When I looked at the films, however, I noted that the shadow was still not seen sharply. Another of my aphorisms was "The purpose of tomograms is to see better," and these were to me unsatisfactory, as they had not accomplished that goal. In fact, I wondered if the shadow was so far forward it might be in the anterior rib rather than the lung.

Musing about the situation, I realized that surely one unusual element of the case was his occupation—a blacksmith. After all, this was in the 1950s, not the 1850s. I asked him where he was employed, and he said at a country club in suburban Westchester County. I asked if no one had commented on his face, and he said he took care to keep it covered. I asked him exactly what a blacksmith did, and he said he took care of the shoeing of the horses, as it was a riding club. A light bulb went off. Were you ever kicked by a horse, I asked? Oh, yes, he remembered, about six months previously a horse had kicked him in the chest while he was shoeing it. He pointed to the spot, just about where the abnormal x-ray shadow was. He had denied injury and had not remembered the incident until specifically asked. I made an unusual order: I had him lie face down on the x-ray table, and I had the tomograms repeated, but now going in the reverse direction, 1, 2 and 3 cm up from the table. Sure enough, the study revealed a fracture of the fifth anterior rib, with healing bone which extended superior to the rib border, making it look like a nodule in the lung! Following my curiosity led to asking the right question, and in turn, to the correct diagnosis.

And I am pleased to say that Moran's face eventually healed after extensive treatment.

Willis Storey offers another relevant example of asking the right questions, but in quite a different circumstance. Storey, twenty-eight years old, had previously experienced a severe closed-head injury, which totally disabled him. Recently he had acutely developed high fever and drenching night sweats. Hospitalized nearby, his x-ray had revealed hundreds of tiny spots evenly distributed throughout his lungs. His physician diagnosed miliary tuberculosis based on the x-ray appearance; "miliary" refers to the spots the size of a type of bird seed. Anti-TB medicines were begun, Storey's temperature subsided, and he was discharged.

To his and his physician's chagrin, his symptoms recurred shortly thereafter—an extremely rare occurrence in TB. Willis was then referred to our hospital. His x-ray did, indeed, show a similar appearance of these recurrent tiny shadows.

We were mystified. I felt certain this was not tuberculosis, so I ordered a battery of sophisticated tests in an attempt to find an alternative diagnosis. Willis was un-communicative; trying to take a complex history from him was difficult. A few days later, however, his wife, a pleasant heavy woman of about the same age, came in to visit, and I was able to talk with her. At one point, curious as to what a disabled unemployed man of twenty-eight did with his time, I asked her just that. "Oh," she said, "he tends to his pigeons." Light bulb again! Storey kept a dovecote on the roof of their apartment. Willis had developed a hypersensitivity, a form of allergy, to his birds; when removed from them during his initial stay at the hospital, his condition had improved; when he returned home, he was re-exposed, and his symptoms had promptly recurred. This pattern is, indeed, typical of what we then called "pigeon breeder's disease." We now know it as a form of hypersensitivity pneumonitis, which involves a reaction to a broad range of inorganic substances.

Inquiring about avocations and hobbies when taking a patient's history is now as fundamental as knowing the patient's occupation itself.

The Director

The consultation from the psychiatric service was not unusual: an abnormal x-ray. Now on staff at the Bronx VA, this was one of my first consultations after returning from the Indian Bureau. I looked at the film. I saw a tiny nodule in the right lung. It was so tiny that you might be surprised it was seen at all, and to me that was important. Nodules which are not particularly dense are hard to distinguish from the surrounding tissues until they reach a moderate size of at least 5 millimeters or so; dense shadows, on the other hand, can be seen even if smaller. This one was not calcified, which would have been an almost absolute sign of benignity, but it was dense enough while so tiny that, once again, a benign situation—the late result of a previous infection—was almost certainly the case. Cancer, as suggested by our radiologist, seemed to me just short of unthinkable. I went to see the patient with a few purposes: to elicit any history suggesting exposure to one of the infections; to make sure there was nothing else in the history or physical exam of concern; to learn if prior x-rays might be available; and to reassure him.

He was a young man in his thirties. He was a movie director, an occupation unusual in our VA population. Originally from the Midwest (where he could have been exposed to the fungus which causes histoplasmosis, a common cause of that type of nodule), he had spent much time in southern California (the same possibility for coccidioidomycosis) and in New York and Europe (the same for tuberculosis). In fact, he had just returned from six months in Copenhagen making a film. Upon return he found his lady friend had run off with another man, leading to the nervous breakdown for which he had been hospitalized.

I found nothing of concern, and began to reassure him. He interrupted. What concerns me, he said, was that he had had a check-up in Copenhagen upon his arrival there, including a chest x-ray, and had been told everything was normal. The nodule must therefore be new, he thought, and perhaps a tumor. I told him the shadow did not look new, but I agreed to attempt to obtain the x-ray, or at least the report, from Copenhagen, and to notify him of the result. My behavior exemplified one of my teaching aphorisms: "There is no substitute for brains, but old films are better."

71

I wrote, and a few weeks later I received a response. The letter started: Dear Herr Doctor Green—not your everyday salutation. The physician went on to say that the x-ray had not been done in his office, but he sent a copy of the report. It read: "Heart normal. In the right lung there is a tiny dense primary healed lesion. The lungs are clear. Impression: normal chest."

I knew nothing, of course, about the experience or competence of the European radiologist, but I was delighted that he or she had agreed with me, even to the extent of not calling the x-ray abnormal. So, as the director's nervous breakdown rapidly resolved, we had a happy outcome all around!

After All, What Else Could It Be?

Sergeant Jimmie Anderson, a twenty-three-year-old black man from North Carolina, was stationed in West Germany. He was "having a ball;" that is, until he started to cough and feel generally ill as spring arrived. Multiple meds prescribed at sick bay didn't help; finally, a chest x-ray was taken. It revealed a 3 cm cavity with surrounding inflammation in the mid-zone of his right lung, strongly suggesting tuberculosis. Anderson was promptly hospitalized on the tuberculosis ward of a major military hospital. No TB germs were found in a smear of his sputum examined under the microscope. This was a bit surprising, but by no means rare; the more definitive test was culture of the sputum. Sadly, this test requires six weeks for completion. More surprising to his physicians was a negative skin test for TB; although this also occurs—rarely— Jimmie seemed to have no reason for his reaction to be suppressed. His physicians reviewed his case: the x-ray and his presentation were so characteristic of TB that they thought that must be the correct diagnosis; after all, what else could it be?

After a short period of study and discussion, Anderson was started on anti-TB medicines. He was transferred back to the States, discharged from the service and admitted to my service at the VA hospital three months later. Fortunately, his records came with him; his cultures for the

TB germ were negative. Unfortunately, in the interim another symptom—severe pain in his right ankle—had developed, and he limped onto the ward. His chest x-ray showed no improvement from his prior ones, but an x-ray of his ankle showed a destructive change in the talus, the bone which connects the leg to the foot. A biopsy of this lesion revealed a fungus infection of the bone, the organism identified as *blastomyces dermatiditis*. We were able to isolate the same germ from his sputum. Anderson had blastomycosis. We stopped his anti-TB medications and started ones aimed at the fungus.

When physicians think "after all, what else can it be," they usually do not ask the question seriously. The lesson here is that they should—there are always other possibilities. A number of fungus diseases, commonly histoplasmosis and blastomycosis, can simulate TB, as they did in Jimmie's case.

But the story does not end there. Surgical stabilization of Anderson's foot was necessary; medical treatment aimed at the fungus continued. After a month a chest x-ray appeared to show some improvement in the cavity, but a new and disturbing finding was present. The lymph glands at the root of the left lung were now swollen. It would surely be unexpected that the disease would simultaneously improve and spread. Could something else be going on? Jimmie's TB skin test was now positive! He had been exposed to and contracted the TB germ while hospitalized among other tuberculous patients. The swollen nodes represented the primary form of tuberculous infection; we recovered the germ from his secretions. It was still susceptible to the anti-TB drugs he had been given, although they clearly had not prevented his infection from progressing to disease (they did not include isoniazid). Eventually both conditions responded well, and Jimmie was discharged.

Bon Mot

Joe Bailey, a forty-two-year-old carpenter, was admitted complaining of a few weeks of a general ill feeling accompanied by fever, cough and headache. On examination his neck appeared to be stiff; his chest x-ray showed areas of spotting in his right upper lung. The combination surely suggested tuberculosis, probably of the lung, and possibly of the meninges, the lining tissues of the brain and spinal cord. The essential diagnostic procedure was a spinal tap for examination of the spinal fluid. His fluid showed the presence of inflammatory cells and increased protein content, and though the reduction in glucose content was slight, these were all compatible with the suspected infection. However, staining for the tuberculosis germ and other germs was negative, as was his sputum exam. As the old saw states, "when you hear hoofbeats, think of horses, not zebras," and tuberculosis was still favored. Tumor was also a possibility.

In the laboratory the technicians performed another examination on the spinal fluid, an India Ink preparation. An organism today named *cryptococcus neoformans*, then more commonly called *Torula histolytica*, is hard to see on routine stains. It has, however, a large fluffy coat: in the presence of India ink, which ordinarily turns the entire field under the microscope dark, the organism's coat does not stain, leaving diagnostic clear zones within the ink. The tech, whose name was Duerr, claimed to have seen these organisms on the smear. Although a rather rare disease in a healthy man, the clinical picture was compatible with cryptococcal meningitis, with involvement of the lung, and this unusual diagnosis (a "zebra") was made.

Bailey's case was promptly selected for presentation at the weekly Medicine conference, where a young radiologist presented the chest x-ray. "You see," he said, "the kind of infiltration seen here is more interstitial than usual, and thus more suggestive of cryptococcosis than tuberculosis." Our pulmonary consultant, Dr. J. Burns Amberson, rose and warned against overuse of vague terms such as interstitial, stating that, in his opinion, the x-ray appearance did not favor one disorder over another.

The denouement? The patient did not improve. A second spinal fluid exam did not show the *Torula* organisms, and shortly thereafter, both the sputum and spinal fluid specimens grew out the tubercle bacillus. The diagnosis was now clearly established as tuberculosis, rather than the less common disorder. The old horses adage—stated another way as, "common diseases are common"—had proved true once again.

The lab tech, Duerr, had certainly made a mistake in the initial interpretation of the India ink preparation. Some grumbling ensued. Fortunately, the error was not fatal, as Bailey gradually responded to treatment for his tuberculosis. As I pointed out at the time: Duerr is human—let's forgive and move on.

What If?

I was furious. What a waste of my time! A patient—himself, a physician—had been admitted to my service prior to his already scheduled transfer to the surgical service. I, a resident internist, was expected to do a physical examination and order routine tests—tasks a capable technician could do, since they required no independent thought whatsoever!

Still fuming, I reviewed the materials in the admission packet. I quickly became absorbed in his history. Dr. England had had a routine check up five years previously, at which time a greatly enlarged heart had been found. Studies at a University center in New York had failed to reveal a cause, but he was told his prognosis was poor with heart failure the likely outcome. Dr. England promptly sold his medical practice and moved to California. Two years later, still alive and well, he was restudied, only to be offered the same diagnosis and prognosis.

An extensive history, taken and retaken, had revealed only two potentially relevant aspects: the first was one minor episode of non-specific chest pain following exertion; the second was an accident he had experienced while in service in North Africa during World War II—he had been thrown out of a jeep and had landed on his chest. An evaluation at the time had shown no damage.

In his prior studies, three further options had been presented to Dr.

England. First was the now standard, but then brand new and considered risky procedure of angiocardiography in which the blood stream is flooded with dye and pictures of the heart and vessels taken. A second option was to tap the pericardial cavity—the space which surrounds the heart—with a needle to determine whether bleeding into that space had occurred after the accident. The third option was surgical exploration and biopsy of the heart. He opted for the last option and returned east for the operation. His surgeon was on the staff of the University hospital, but he was also a consultant at the VA, which is why he was admitted here.

On exam I found a pleasant man, anxious to move ahead. His heart sounds seemed soft and distant to me, but otherwise normal. I ordered a battery of routine tests. His electrocardiogram showed "low voltage," a non-specific finding. Blood counts and chemistries were normal. For the chest x-ray our hospital had recently inaugurated a routine of adding a view from the side, a lateral view. The report noted the enlarged heart in the frontal view, but in the lateral, the radiologist saw a suggestion of gas bubbles, air-filled structures, just under the breast bone. A flurry of excitement led to abdominal x-ray studies which revealed a most remarkable finding: a large portion of the colon was present in his chest! Surgery revealed more exactly that the transvese colon was literally within the pericardial space. In the jeep accident the force of the fall had apparently ruptured the diaphragm—the muscle which separates the chest and abdominal contents—permitting the bizarre herniation. The heart itself was entirely normal. The colon was replaced, and the defect repaired.

Most astonishing was the fact that, during the five years of this anatomic rearrangement, Dr. England had experienced no gastrointestinal complications. The multiple "what if" scenarios became the source of jocund speculation. What if an intestinal growl, heard while the chest was being examined, had been interpreted as a bizarre cardiac murmur? What if he had developed diverticulitis? The biggest laugh came from imagining the look on the examiner's face, if, when he had attempted aspiration of the pericardial space, his needle recovered feces instead of fluid!

In addition to his eventual recovery, there were two other positive outcomes. Dr. England quickly resumed his practice. And my case report of his condition and findings became my first scientific publication.

The Indian Bureau

Culture Shock

First Assignment

When I entered the Indian Bureau in January 1952, I felt prepared for experiences with the different cultures I would undoubtedly meet. I felt receptive, perhaps better fit than many, for the issues which I might have to face. My Jewish background, as a member of a "different" culture, was partially responsible, as was my general level of education and sensitivity. Furthermore, I had an interest in cultural anthropology. In the summer of 1946, my first summer out of uniform after the war, between my second and third years of medical school, I had even taken a summer course at Columbia University in the subject, where I absorbed the works of Margaret Mead, Ralph Linton, Ruth Benedict and others. I was ready for the experience. Or so I thought.

My first assignment was at the Indian Tuberculosis Sanatorium in Albuquerque, New Mexico. I was to assist Dr. Robert Saylor, a long time Indian Bureau tuberculosis physician. Most of the patients at the Albuquerque San were members of the dozen or so various Pueblo tribes, which led to my first surprising experience. The first weekend I was on duty covering the sanatorium, I was called in because a fight had broken out on the male ward. It was between a Zuni Indian and an Apache from

77

the Mescalero area over some apparently trivial food-related matter. Fortunately it had ended before I arrived. A discussion followed between the combatants and a group of a dozen or so others. I was impressed with one speaker, the brother of the Zuni man, who spoke in a sophisticated universalist tone about utilization of the resources of the hospital. The speech was very powerful. Then he concluded: "Yes," he said, "I think everybody should be able to come here—of course, as long as he is an Indian." The we/they dichotomy I had seen elsewhere was as prevalent here as anywhere; just the specific classes were new to me.

A significant group of the patients, indeed the largest single group, was Navajo. One of the first patients I helped care for was Mary Lee, a pathetically wasted young woman with far advanced disease. She breathed shallowly and painfully and was clearly terminal, as was not unusual in those days. To my shock and surprise, Dr. Saylor gave permission to her family for her to leave the sanatorium and be taken back to the reservation for a "sing." As I understood it, this ritual of Navajo medicine included an elaborate sand painting (using sands of different colors) made by a Navajo healer. There were chants, prayers, and a gathering of the families—a kind of pre-death service. These patients were, themselves, highly contagious; so it surprised me that Dr. Saylor would send them home to die and, in doing so, expose others—particularly the next generation—to the disease. In retrospect, I realized I exaggerated the danger. Most of the relatives had been infected previously; nevertheless, I was worried about the youngsters for whom this might be the infecting incident. I understood Dr. Saylor's attitude, but I had some trouble agreeing with it.

Another patient with active TB was a sad-faced little Navaho girl about nine years old named Lyda Joe. She spoke little English and seemed uncommunicative. I was told her parents were dead, and that she had been brought to the san and dumped there by her grandfather. It appeared that all she had done in her young life was tend to a flock of sheep. She had not been to school, and details about the rest of her life were unknown. She had advanced tuberculosis of a type that was unusual for children and more often seen in adults. In the sanatorium, rest, good food, anti tuberculosis medications and a supportive environment worked semi-wonders. Lyda Joe gained weight, learned a bit of English, began to smile and relate to the staff and other children. Her progress brought great satisfaction to everyone who knew her.

After three months in Albuquerque, I had a call from the central office of the Public Health Service in Washington. I was asked to temporarily be in charge of the Tuberculosis division at the Indian Bureau Medical Center in Talihina, far away in southeastern Oklahoma. The position was vacant after the unexpected death of the hospital director, who had had some experience with TB. My wife and I packed a few belongings, closed our rental apartment, and left for what we thought would be a short excursion. After three months in Talihina I decided to stay on, relishing the opportunity to be in charge of the sanatorium. We returned to Albuquerque to pack up and say goodbye.

At the san, Dr Saylor's disappointment with my decision to leave was evident. We talked about a number of patients, and then I asked about Lyda, never anticipating his heartbreaking response. Shortly after I had left, her grandfather had appeared at the sanatorium, apparently wondering why he had not heard about her death. When he saw her and she looked "well," he immediately took her back to the reservation to resume her life tending his sheep. The staff pleaded with him to let her stay, but to no avail. They knew her leaving meant she would rapidly worsen and die, but there was nothing anyone could do. Perhaps unfairly, I ascribed his selfish, unsympathetic behavior both before and after her hospitalization to his culture. He may just have been a mean, old man. The experience left me with a deep distress I feel to this day.

In Talihina

One of the first patients I admitted after my arrival in Talihina was Philip Bear. He was an eighteen-year-old Creek, a good looking young man. A year previously his draft board had rejected him for service because of an abnormal chest x-ray, which he did not follow up on. Now he was brought to our hospital almost terminally ill by his family, who then departed. Both lungs were heavily involved, particularly the right upper lobe, where he had a thick-walled cavity. In addition, he had scrofula—draining tuberculous lymph nodes in his neck. His prognosis was poor. In the days before chemotherapy he surely would have died. Because of the long distances between a patient's home and the sanatorium, and the inability of these poor people to travel easily, it was our custom to have a blank consent form signed for minors before the family left in the event emergency surgery was required. This behavior was not strictly legal, but we felt it necessary and the best we could do under the circumstances. Philip's family had signed the form.

After three months, when I reviewed his progress, to my surprise and pleasure, Philip was doing very well. His neck was healing; he had gained twenty pounds from fewer than 100 pounds; his left lung was clearing nicely, and it looked as if the main problem would be that right upper lobe. I wrote an informative letter to his family, who lived in Oklahoma City, and told them he had improved, and that I might wish to do a thoracoplasty—surgery to remove the ribs over the cavity so it could close and heal—if he continued to do well. I received no answer. After another three months, further significant clearing had occurred around the cavity, and Philip looked like a healthy young man. I wrote again. In the early days of chemotherapy we did not know how long-lasting the improvement might be, and we still considered the addition of older methods of care reasonable. I said that the deforming surgery might not be necessary, and that I might wish instead to do a pneumothorax—a temporary procedure that could later be reversed without any permanent damage. Although I had a consent on file, I was uncomfortable proceeding with it; I asked for their consent.

My wife and I lived on the grounds in a three-bedroom native stone house adjacent to the hospital. Newspapers were delivered for all of our compound at the hospital lobby. It was a Sunday morning. Still in my robe, before breakfast, I went over to get the Sunday paper. There was an old Indian man sitting in the lobby, dressed in a mechanic's uniform. It was Philip Bear's father. He was clearly a cut above many of my usual patients and their families, both in education and income. He said he had come because of my letter and asked about it. I took him into the x-ray room, pulled all of Philip's films, and went over the case with him, as if he were a colleague (which, of course, he was, in the sense of both of us caring for Philip). I finished my presentation. I asked if he would sign consent for the pneumothorax.

He paused, and then said, "No, I think I will take him home."

I was stunned. "Take him home!?"

"Yes," he said.

"Why?" I asked. He shook his head and mumbled under his breath. I persisted: "Don't you think we have done well by him here?"

"No, he doesn't look particularly different to me"—this about a boy who had gained fifty pounds.

"And he is still not well," I said.

"Well," he said, "we have doctors too." (He was referring to Indian doctors—herb doctors, native practitioners with no medical training.) I was aghast. I became very upset—in part for Philip, but more, I think, because I was angry and frustrated by my own inability to communicate adequately with him, to convince him, to make him see that I cared, and that I knew what was right for Philip. I was young, twenty-seven, and not a model of aequinimatas. My voice rose along with my despair and concern. Suddenly, he stopped, put his head backward and upright, as if withdrawing a step, and laughed.

"What are you laughing at?" I burst out.

"Never saw a white man get upset about an Indian before," he said. As far as he was concerned, my entire behavior was obviously ridiculous, incomprehensible to him, an unreal act. I believe the history of prior racism to which he was accustomed took precedence over me as an individual who really cared for his son.

Philip left with his father. After my service in the Indian Bureau had ended and I had returned to New York, I learned that Philip had later been brought back to the sanatorium in terrible condition and had died.

Living in Oklahoma provided me with another cultural experience about prejudice. In most of the Western United States, including New Mexico, at that time most of the white population looked down upon the Indians as an inferior race. The same was true in the South, where the indigenous Native Americans had been shipped to Indian Territory in the early 19th century. But not so in Oklahoma, where the reverse was true. Perhaps because Indian Territory became most of the state, most Oklahomans I met were proud if they had any Indian blood and would openly boast about it. This seemed to apply to just about everyone in Talihina. Sadly though, that part of the state was called "Little Dixie," and everybody looked down on the few Negroes there. It was a confirming lesson for me that the expression of prejudice, at least in part, is dependent upon local attitudes and upbringing.

Good, Wholesome Food

One aspect of culture shock has an amusing side to it. In 1952 the Bureau of Indian Affairs was within the administration of the Department of the Interior (having been transferred there from the Department of War (!) years before). As the Public Health Service gradually began to assume responsibility for staffing the Bureau, additional health professionals began to arrive in Talihina. One of these was Betty Lasker, a trained and certified nutritionist, originally from New York. I'm not certain who had chosen the menus prior to her arrival, but sanatorium meals seemed at least adequate, helped along by a good supply of local vegetables. Betty immediately began what she considered a more scientific approach to the diets.

Meat had been somewhat of a problem in the sanatorium. Pork, the meat staple for the Oklahoma Indians, was fortunately readily available. To the transplanted Navajos, on the other hand, lamb or mutton was desirable; the local Indians found it unappetizing, to say the least. Betty was unaware of these difficulties. To her what counted was the nutritional value of the food itself. For her, there was no doubt that the ideal food was beef. So a few weeks after her arrival, at considerable additional expense, a handsome beef dinner was served to the resident patients. Something, finally, united the culinary tastes of the two groups: nobody found the beef palatable, and nobody ate it! Betty learned the hard way that there's more to successful nutrition than merely determining intrinsic food values.

My Obstetric Practice

First Delivery

We arrived at the Talihina Medical Center, presumably on temporary duty, in April 1952. Two other doctors were on staff there: the acting Director, a general practitioner who was also the surgeon, and a second GP. I was in charge of the 160-bed sanatorium portion, and they took care of the 90-bed general hospital. With only three doctors available, however, it was understood that we shared call—every third night. That was fine with me.

A week or so later Miss Oberholzer, one of the nurses, called me at home at about 10:00 p.m. It was the proverbial dark and stormy night, complete with thunder, lightning and heavy rain. From my door to the hospital entrance was just about twenty yards, and I went directly to the labor/delivery suite on the second floor. Miss Oberholzer was taking care of a young Indian woman, in her mid-twenties, unmarried, in labor with her first child. She was a big woman, tall, broad and heavy, though not fat.

I entered with some trepidation. In Medical School our practical obstetric experience was on what was called 24-hour OB. On call to go anywhere in the city when a woman was in labor, I had delivered three—and only three—black babies in their homes on the south side of Chicago. Our team had consisted of another medical student and a nurse midwife. I did not then question the concept or ethics of home delivery by an inexperienced medical student. After all, these were poor people, who could not afford much in the way of medical care; they were fortunate to have any health professional at all there for the home delivery. I was thankful that the three deliveries went well, with healthy mothers and babies. Oddly, this had been the very last two-week rotation of my senior year, and I did not feel I had exactly mastered obstetrics. My rotating internship at Mt. Sinai Hospital in New York City was in striking contrast. I had no obstetrical experience there whatsoever—interns were not thought mature or knowledgeable enough to care for pregnant patients in the private pavilion. In retrospect, I am amazed that I just accepted these remarkable inequalities in access to health care; it

83

surely was a different time. In any case, as I entered the labor room in Talihina, there awaited my fourth delivery.

The woman seemed to be in hard labor. By rectal exam I could tell that the cervix was fully dilated, but after an hour or so nothing seemed to be happening, despite regular hard contractions. I called the surgeon's house and spoke to him. He thought I should just be patient, not offering to come in himself. Meanwhile the storm raged outside. After continued lack of progress, I took a look inside the vagina. A large soft bluish bag bulged at me. I assumed it was the amniotic sac—the bag of waters. I asked Miss Oberholzer if the doctors here would puncture the bag to release the waters to help the delivery along, as I remembered from medical school, and she said they did. I took a clamp and grasped the bag. To my surprise and distress, no fluid exuded; instead, it was tissue, and when I pinched it, it bled. It was the placenta, not the bag of waters, and it was oozing blood. *Placenta previa*, the condition when the placenta presents before the child, is a dangerous situation, threatening both the mother and the child with death. I called the surgeon, told him what had happened and asked him to come in. Once again, this time to my distress, he just told me to be patient, and hung up.

The very difficult labor continued. When the baby's head appeared, it presented posteriorly, referring to the position of the head coming down the birth canal. This is the reverse of the usual presentation, and more dangerous. But luck was with me and with all of us: the story ends with the baby finally being born, and born healthy; the mother did not bleed excessively, the placenta separated normally, and just before dawn I went home. And there concluded my obstetric baptism under fire. The truth of the old aphorism was proved again—it is better to be lucky than smart—or experienced—or competent!

Babies, babies, babies

All in all, I delivered 102 babies in Talihina—and none since. Although a bit nervous at first, I gradually gained confidence with each successful delivery. The vast majority of my patients were young healthy

Choctaw women, and most of the deliveries went smoothly. And to my pleasure—and surprise—even the somewhat more complex ones went well. Fortunately, I never had to deal with any life-threatening problems. Most of the deliveries were without incident, but some, in addition to that first one, are worthy of remembering.

Louise Pickup, a Creek Indian, was twenty-three when she was admitted with tuberculosis in her left lung plus surrounding pleural fluid. She was two months pregnant with her first child. I started her antituberculosis medications, including the new agent isoniazid; she did well. The baby, however, a breech presentation, was stillborn at birth, with large polycystic kidneys. I wrote to a friend and consultant at the Mayo Clinic, who was keeping a registry, to inquire whether or not the drug could have been responsible. He said they had no knowledge of isoniazid being harmful during pregnancy. Based on much scientific data, that remains the opinion even today, but I couldn't help wondering about it then, and still do.

This next experience is a bit unpleasant, so you might want to skip reading it if you are squeamish. We all knew about the Rh factor then, but did not test for it routinely. You will recall that if a mother is Rh negative, and the baby Rh positive, the mother can develop antibodies which can severely impact the fetus. One night on call, I delivered a young woman after great difficulty. The baby was stillborn and monstrously swollen. It had fetal hydrops, erythroblastosis fetalis, the Rh factor disease—but her tests, subsequently performed, showed no Rh abnormality. This was a long time ago, and we knew little about other blood factors that could be responsible for the syndrome. While attending to the mother postpartum, we had placed the stillborn infant in a large basin on its stomach. Afterwards when I examined it more carefully, the pressure from the basin had actually obliterated its facial features. Quite sad.

Mary Ann Knight, a Cherokee woman, had had at least a dozen prior pregnancies and known chronic tuberculosis for two years. (One of her babies had, itself, died of TB.) This time I admitted her to the sanatorium at about seven month's gestation. Her abdomen was remarkably pendulous, and when she stood, the upside-down pregnant uterus, and the large baby it held, literally hung down to her knees! I

85

was quite concerned about the delivery, because of her lax abdominal wall, the bizarre position of the uterus and my fear that the uterine wall was abnormally stretched and thinned. But I needn't have been worried; when she went into labor, she essentially gave one or two big pushes and out came a fourteen-pound viable healthy girl!

Another night, I was called in to deliver a Choctaw woman, who had had seven prior deliveries, all girls. This time I delivered a boy. When I told her with great excitement that she had a son, she seemed surprisingly subdued for such news. I asked why. She told me that her husband had performed the Choctaw ring test, and that they already knew the baby was a boy. In their version of the test, when the mother feels the baby has begun kicking, the husband suspends her wedding ring on a long string over the mother's abdomen: if the ring just hangs there passively, the baby will be a girl; if the ring spins around actively, it will be a boy. She claimed that for all seven prior pregnancies the ring test had correctly predicted a girl. This time, when it indicated a boy, the entire family held their big celebration prior to the actual delivery. I wondered what might have happened if it had been another girl! The "test," or something like it, is apparently not limited to Native American cultures; an example among the Greeks can be found in the recent novel *Middlesex* by Jeffrey Eugenides.

Betty Foster, a half-blooded Cherokee woman, was thirty-two when admitted. She had had TB for five years, never completely controlled. When I saw Betty, her right upper lobe was destroyed and shrunken; she also had a large cavity in the right lower lobe. I started medications and instituted pneumoperitoneum. In this procedure great volumes of air are instilled into the abdominal cavity to apply upward pressure on the diaphragm and the lungs above them, which hopefully then relax and, thereby, heal. (A side benefit of the procedure was my ability to see the outline of the upper abdominal organs, the liver and the spleen.) Betty started to improve, but after a month or so began to have vaginal spotting unrelated, she said, to her menses. I examined her and thought I felt a mass on her left side in the region of her Fallopian tube and ovary. I then had what I thought was a brilliant idea. I turned her upside down on a tilting x-ray table and took an x-ray in this position. I reasoned that the intraabdominal air would now rise into her pelvis, which was now superior, and might outline the mass I had felt. The air did rise, as expected, but all I saw was a shadow in the midline and no mass. Oh well, I thought, another apparently creative idea down the drain. Then, a month later, Betty spontaneously aborted a three month fetus. The midline shadow I had noted was the enlarged uterus, so my idea was not so crackpot after all!

One humorous anecdote related to Betty's recovery. One day that summer, my wife Lila was home and heard a knock at the door. When she opened it, a man, apparently a farmer, stood there. Lila, a young and beautiful twenty-three, was probably wearing shorts and some kind of short top, making her look even younger. "Is this Dr. Green's house?" he asked.

"Yes."

"Is your father home?"

After Lila's identity was cleared up, the man said, "I'm Foster. This is for you." He then handed her a big basket of vegetables, fresh from his farm. Betty had apparently spoken of her doctor in positive terms; Betty's husband must have assumed I was older than a man in his twenties. The gift was in gratitude for my care. Lila and I eventually laughed about the assumptions patients can make about the age and appearance of doctors and their families. We blamed Hollywood for reflecting the stereotypes and prejudices of American society.

Now do you believe it?

One afternoon a woman brought her teenage daughter to our clinic because of abdominal pain. The pain was cramping in nature, had started the previous day, and hadn't responded to a laxative. The physician on duty took one look at the fifteen-year-old and announced that she was in labor. The mother said, "Don't be ridiculous, my daughter can't even be pregnant."

They argued about it, but then my colleague noted the girl beginning to grunt and push with each frequent pain. He put the girl on a stretcher and rang for our slow elevator to take her to the delivery room on the second floor. Too late: with the mother still in complete denial, he delivered the baby right there on the elevator. He held the baby up by its heels and shouted at the mother, "Now do you believe it?"

We all laughed about the situation later on, though we realized it was also a sad commentary on a local situation. The religious orientation of many of the local residents was such that drinking, smoking, dating, dancing, movies and most every form of relaxation were forbidden for their children. It was not surprising to us that teenage pregnancy was fairly common.

Panic

Perhaps my most unusual obstetric experience occurred one summer weekend. Some of my friends in town, including Doc Johnson, an osteopathic general physician and the only private physician in the area, had invited me to go to St. Louis with them to see the Brooklyn Dodgers play the Cardinals. I was on call, and so declined. The next night I received a phone call from a local young white farmer, Buddy Edwards. He said his wife was in labor with their first child, but he couldn't find Doc Johnson (I knew exactly where he was!). Could he bring her to the Hospital? The Indian Hospital was restricted to Indian patients, but an emergency is an emergency, so I said of course.

I met Mrs. Edwards at the hospital. She was a pretty blond woman in advanced, active labor. I admitted her directly to the delivery room. Everything seemed to be going smoothly. When I actually delivered the baby boy, however, I was shocked: he had a strange deathly white pallor! Reflexly, my first thought was *"asphyxia pallida."* (When a newborn is oxygen starved, it may show discoloration of two types: commonly, a grayish-blue, called *"asphyxia livida,"* or a rarer and more serious lack of color, *"asphyxia pallida."* The latter term describes a pre-birth illness, which ordinarily predicts a seriously ill or even dead infant.) My mind raced with instantaneous panic: this child has *asphyxia pallida*!! Yet this baby was squalling, and kicking, and moving around vigorously. I finally realized (this all taking place in a matter of seconds) that the "problem" with the child was: *it was white*! Up to now, I had been delivering only dusky, healthy, reddish dark-skinned Indian babies, and the contrast with this blond Caucasian infant was startling!

Everything happily resolved, as mother, father, baby—and doctor—relaxed and did well.

Doctoring

While in Talihina, I particularly enjoyed the opportunity to practice general medicine. I was, after all, the primary physician for the ills of a large group of people, who just happened to have tuberculosis; I also was on call at the general hospital clinic and wards, where I continued to learn some striking lessons.

First Victory

'Fair is foul, and foul is fair:
Hover through the fog and filthy air.'
Macbeth

The morning after we arrived in Talihina I was taken around the hospital for a general tour. At one point during the tour, when we were starting up the steps to the second floor of the men's tuberculosis ward, I was hit with a foul odor permeating the staircase. It was the very typical foul odor of anaerobic infection, of putrefaction, of a lung abscess—infection with certain specific bacteria, usually caused by aspiration of infected material from the upper airway into the lungs. The smell was coming from the first room next to the stairway, as far as possible from the nurse's station and the other patients. The man in the room was lying there, stuporous, though he smiled when aroused. This was clearly going to be the first case to require my immediate attention.

Lemos Goings, forty-three, a full-blooded Choctaw man, had come to the hospital the prior summer with cough and chest pain. His x-ray showed some suspicious shadows in the left lower lobe, but his sputum was negative for TB. They did note he had severe dental pyorrhea. Their diagnosis was stable TB; he was discharged without any treatment. In December he returned. He had been deteriorating, and his sputum was foul. Now his x-ray showed dense disease involving most of the left lower chest. A tap to check for pleural fluid was negative. He received streptomycin, which treats general infection as well as TB, for some months, and some penicillin and aureomycin (a popular broad spectrum antibiotic of that time), all to no avail. I examined him promptly. His story, particularly with the foul sputum and clubbing of his digits, made the diagnosis of anaerobic infection with or without an abscess, clear-cut. I began treatment with high dose penicillin. I also had the nurses give him oxygen to breathe—it's an old trick which rapidly cleanses the foulness of the sputum—and I became a hero to the staff. Not bad for my first week there!

Lemos cleared up mentally, and despite his limited English, turned into a jovial and responsive man. He gained thirty pounds. His x-ray cleared with some residual large areas of destruction in the lower lobe (which, in fact, were reinfected later after I left). I discharged him after a few months. Lemos Goings was one of my earliest triumphs in Talihina. It surely was the quickest way to gain the immediate respect for my ability from the nursing staff!

If It Ain't Broke

The Talihina Medical Center was a single, beautiful, native stone hospital building when I arrived in 1952. It had two main sections: in the front were the administrative offices and two general hospital floors, each with forty beds, also including an operating room and an obstetrical suite. A long corridor leading to the rear contained the laboratories, radiology division and the tuberculosis treatment rooms. And, to the rear, were the tuberculosis wards: four wards on two floors, each with forty beds. The tuberculosis division was my responsibility; however, when

I arrived, only two other physicians covered the general hospital. We arranged it so that each of the three of us would be on call, by rotation, on nights and weekends.

My first night on call I made a quick rounds with the nursing staff on the general floors. I wanted to familiarize myself with the system and get a passing acquaintance with the patients then hospitalized, especially those acutely ill. As I went by one of the single rooms, I saw a scrawny, elderly man lying quietly. The nurse told me, "Oh, that's Mr. Kelly. He has terminal stomach cancer." I thought nothing more about it as we continued rounds.

As the months went by, I settled into a comfortable routine during my nights on call. If there were no new patients arriving in clinic, or no hospitalized ones requiring specific attention, I would do my familiarizing rounds, then return to my house on the hospital grounds to await any call from the nurses.

I don't recall exactly how long it took, but one night I realized I had been passing by Mr. Kelly's room for many, many months, and by all appearances, he seemed unchanged in all that time. I was surprised that, given terminal cancer, he was still alive. I picked up his chart for review. He had been admitted almost a year before, complaining of abdominal pain, loss of appetite and weight loss, certainly symptoms suggestive of his diagnosis. The admitting physician had also drawn a sketch in the chart of his physical findings: a large mass filling the central upper portion of his abdomen. It had been decided these findings were adequate for the diagnosis. No further studies had been done, as his general state precluded the possibility of surgery. Kelly had received supportive care and, otherwise, had been basically ignored.

I decided to check the physical findings for myself. A cancerous mass should surely have progressed. The mass I felt, however, was about the same size as the drawing in the chart; but more important, it was pulsatile! With each beat of the heart, I felt the same beat in the mass. It was possible that a malignancy had attached itself to the aorta, the major blood vessel carrying blood to the lower half of the body, which lay just behind the stomach; but, in view of his indolent course, it seemed a much more likely diagnosis was an aneurysm—a weakening of the wall, coupled with a major enlargement—of the aorta. Although this would be a serious condition in its own right, Kelly's prognosis would surely be better than if he had had advanced stomach cancer.

I re-drew the picture and recorded my reasoning and diagnosis in the chart. This simple act created a flurry of activity the next day. Far from being ignored, Kelly was reexamined extensively by the other physicians as well as the nurses. "Well, whaddya know!" type comments were heard throughout the hospital. The attitude of benign neglect transformed to one of active interest. Unfortunately, should the new diagnosis be confirmed, no surgical approach was available at that time, even if his general condition had permitted it. But it was hoped Kelly could be encouraged to be more active and even discharged.

It was not to be. Two days after the change in diagnosis and the increased attention, Kelly was found in his room, lifeless. His abdomen was markedly swollen; the aneurysm had burst. He had bled massively into his abdominal cavity and died of the hemorrhage and the shock. Had my intervention proved fatal? Perhaps the increased attention to the mass and the multiple physical examinations it had undergone contributed to the rupture. It is impossible to say, as rupture is the natural outcome for many large aneurysms. It might well have ruptured anyway without any provocation. Nevertheless, I felt my investigation surely had not helped! When things are going well, often the best approach is to leave well enough alone.

Obviously, this principle can easily be carried too far. If one took it literally in all situations, there would be no such thing as preventive medicine, and asymptomatic patients with potential life-threatening conditions would go uninvestigated. Some clear-cut examples would include the woman with a painless lump in her breast, or the man with a nodule on a routine chest x-ray. Still, it is a principle worth keeping in mind.

And yet, many years later I seemed to have forgotten it.

In the middle of my career as a pulmonary specialist, I took a detour into medical administration. For eleven years I was an Associate Dean at our medical school. During that time I spent a few hours a week—not very much, it is true—participating in the clinical activities of my division in an attempt to keep up to date. Shortly after I returned full time to my pulmonary practice, I noticed an elderly man with a cane who, every now and then, would limp past my office, and then a few hours later, would limp back. It eventually entered my consciousness that this round trip had been going on for quite some time, and I had no idea what it was all about!

Out of curiosity I finally decided to check. At that time we were participating in a multicenter study of chemotherapy for lung cancer. The office and treatment room of the fellow handling the day-to-day affairs of that program were down the hall past my office. So in one sense I was not surprised to learn that the patient, one Noel Stevens, was in that program. But I realized that Stevens had been making this trek for over a year. I checked his records further. A man with severe, albeit stable, coronary heart disease, he had been admitted originally with symptoms of pneumonia in the left lower lobe of his lung. It had failed to respond promptly to treatment; bronchoscopy, a procedure in which a lighted tube was passed into the lungs to inspect the bronchi, had been performed. The bronchus to the left lower lobe was abnormal: it appeared twisted, scarred and thickened. Specimens from it were taken by biopsy; under the microscope the cells were abnormal, crushed and angry looking. The changes were strongly suspicious of cancer. The pathologist was unwilling to make this diagnosis from the tissue biopsy, as the specimen was too distorted; however, another test—the Papanicolau smear technique—revealed a few malignant cells, and lung cancer was diagnosed.

Extensive studies showed no spread of the tumor outside the chest; however, Stevens was in no condition for curative surgery. He was offered the opportunity to participate in the research study, which included the options of radiation and drugs. He consented. His medication—a chemical agent given intravenously in recurrent cycles—was to continue until relapse occurred. Over the time I had seen him passing by my office, his condition had remained stable.

I reviewed all Stevens's records and materials. His course and his x-rays, including some sophisticated studies, had remained unchanged all that time. In view of the somewhat shaky nature of the original diagnosis, I asked for a thorough review of the early materials, which concluded that the diagnosis was questionable. As continued exposure to the potentially toxic chemotherapy agent could be hazardous, I felt bronchoscopy was again in order to see if evidence of cancer could be confirmed in the diseased left lower lobe. It was performed; multiple biopsies and washings were done. After careful review, it was decided that, although atypical cells were noted, they were not only inadequate to establish the cancer diagnosis, but that they were also very similar to the cells upon which the original diagnosis had been based. Noel may never had had cancer; in any case, it would seem reasonable that his chemotherapy could be discontinued.

It was not to be. That night, a few hours after the procedure, Stevens spiked a temperature to 103 degrees; infection was suspected; cultures of his blood were taken and antibiotics begun, but an hour later a cardiac arrhythmia—an abnormal heart beat—led to a cardiac arrest from which, even though he was in the hospital and advanced life support techniques were rapidly applied, Stevens failed to recover.

The question again hits hard. Had I not attempted to investigate and correct a possible incorrect diagnosis and treatment, would Stevens have continued to walk regularly past my office door for an indefinite period? I cannot help but feel that I should have left well enough alone.

I Never Thought of It!

I admitted Steve Morris, a twenty-seven-year-old, full-blooded Choctaw, in the fall of 1952. He had been acutely ill for a week with chills and fever, headache and mental cloudiness, followed by shortness of breath and chest pain. He had been hospitalized for TB twice before: at age nineteen, for eleven months, for "a spot on the lung," and then for a month at age twenty-four at the Shawnee sanatorium, where a gastric culture was said to be positive. With this past history, he came directly to the TB ward.

His chest x-ray showed some scarring in both upper lobes and a diffuse haze over the right lower two-thirds of the chest, which I thought was either a pleural effusion, pleural reaction or even maybe a pulmonary shadow. I thought his acute illness unlikely to be TB (his smears and later cultures were negative) and promptly started him on penicillin. There was no response, his confusion and unremitting high temperature continuing. A spinal tap was negative. His white blood cell counts, surprisingly, were low—4700 and 5600. I switched to terramycin—still no response. Looking for something unusual, I questioned him more closely and found he had recently hunted, killed and skinned rabbits. I wrote a note in the chart: "History, severe illness, typhoidal mental state, and failure to respond suggest tularemia," although in tularemia the white count is usually high. I sent off serum for serologic tests—agglutination reactions—to the state laboratory. I started streptomycin, and his temperature appeared to respond. On the next day his serological studies were reported: tularemia negative—but the typhoid antigens were highly positive! The diagnosis was typhoid fever, which despite my note about the typhoidal mental state I had never considered. In one day Steve responded to chloramphenicol, the most specific agent for typhoid fever then available, cleared mentally, and developed a voracious appetite. The effusion, or whatever, resolved.

As he was improving, his wife arrived. She was a large healthy appearing woman. I said: "Your husband doesn't appear to have active TB, but he does have an unusual serious illness called typhoid fever."

"Oh, I know about that," she said. "I had it three years ago!" It was likely he had contracted the disease from her, although she refused the studies that would have proved she was a typhoid carrier.

Morris's titers—the level of his blood antibodies—rose and then fell. He left the sanatorium against advice before I could decide whether or not he needed treatment for TB. In his chart I wrote, "If he returns to clinic, be sure and get serology." He did return—and whoever saw him ordered a serologic test for syphilis which, truth be told, was usually what was meant by the non-specific term "serology." I had carelessly not been specific enough. About a year after that he did return with an injured knee, and his titers had fallen to near normal.

Incidentally, prior to Morris I had never seen an actual case of typhoid fever, but I saw a half dozen more in Talihina, and became quite adept at the clinical diagnosis.

My Non Nobel

Dr. John Sutherland, a physician who won recognition for innovative use of biochemical drugs on chronic psychiatric patients, (has) died. Working as a principal research scientist at the Rockland Psychiatric Center in Orangeburg, N. Y. in the 1950's, Dr. Sutherland observed the euphoric effects of a certain drug type on tuberculosis patients. Work then began to find out whether the compound could help hospital patients with severe chronic depression. The experiments with the substance—iproniazid, from a class now identified as monoamine oxidase inhibitors—succeeded. The findings were described in 1957.

New York Times, March 29, 2001, p. A22

When I arrived at the Talihina Medical Center in April 1952, *LIFE* magazine had just published the first public report on the use of two new anti-tuberculosis drugs, rimifon and marsilid, known generically as isoniazid and iproniazid. The report included photos of patients at Sea View Hospital on Staten Island dancing in the corridors of the wards. In my mind, such a euphoric reaction among these patients was not surprising. After months—and often years—of chronic listlessness, fatigue, malaise, fever, cough, blood spitting, and hopeless illness—to suddenly experience marked improvement would naturally create a new overwhelming feeling of well being. Other Indian Bureau physicians with whom I spoke confirmed the same miraculous results in their own experience with patients. Dr. Saylor was impressed with it. One side effect, he noted, was the tremendous appetite patients developed. He feared hypoglycemia—low blood sugar—if they were not given whatever they wanted to eat in whatever quantities. He told me, for example, that a patient I had known in Albuquerque had to have twelve eggs each day for breakfast, or else he complained bitterly of being unsatiated.

We now know the increased appetite was real, but it was due to the euphoric feeling of well being experienced by the patients when their condition improved after being chronically ill for years.

Both isoniazid and iproniazid appeared to be equally effective against tuberculosis, but isoniazid seemed to have a better safety profile, and so it rapidly became the favored agent. I received my own supply of the drug shortly after reading the *LIFE* magazine article. It was a small supply, so I carefully chose which patients would be treated with it. But I also considered two other possibilities to explain the euphoric effects the patients were experiencing. The first was that the euphoria was perhaps evidence of a kind of mass hysteria; and the second was that it might be a nonspecific chemical psychiatric effect—a result of direct action of the drug on the brain, having nothing to do with its effect on the tuberculosis or the patient's reaction to it.

Cancer was rare in my Indian patients, but at the time a man in our hospital was dying with widespread kidney cancer. He was as miserable, if not more so, than my tuberculous patients, although he had not been as ill for as long. I had carefully husbanded my meager supply of drug, but I decided to treat him with the precious medicine, in the same dosage as my TB patients (100 mgm three times a day) to see what effect, if any, it would have. He showed absolutely no response whatsoever. Even though I knew one patient did not represent an adequate experiment, it seemed clear to me that the behavior of the tuberculous patients was related to the response of their tuberculosis, and not an effect of the drug on the brain. So that was that.

As it turned out, the agent I had received was isoniazid, not iproniazid, and it was iproniazid that Sutherland, Kline and others had found to be an effective psychiatric drug.

So, in the exaggerated annals of what might have been, that explains why I didn't win the Nobel—or any—prize!

Summer

One warm afternoon in the summer of 1953 I was in clinic when a mother brought in her sturdy seven-year-old Choctaw boy named Reed. He had been complaining of pain in his legs, which had worsened over the last few days. Now he wouldn't walk. She was understandably concerned. The boy lay stretched out on the examining cot and, indeed, he wasn't moving much. I examined him: he did not flinch or complain of tenderness when I squeezed his thigh and leg muscles. Both of his knees were swollen, very tender, and felt warmer than the surrounding tissues. His right wrist was similar. She told me that, in fact, he had complained of his wrists being sore a few days previously. His joints, not his muscles, seemed to be the source of the distress. She also recalled, in response to my direct questioning, that he had seemed to have had a bad cold with a sore throat earlier in the month.

I had already noted Reed's pulse rate was rapid. With some trepidation I examined his heart: it was enlarged to my percussion note. And when I listened, his heart rate was fast, but despite the rapidity, I could hear a third sound, so that the rhythm resembled a gallop. I also noted irregularities in the beat and a loud persistent murmur.

I felt pretty sure of my diagnosis. I turned to the boy's mother and told her I thought he had acute rheumatic fever. She breathed an audible sigh of apparent relief, and said, "Thank God! I was afraid it was polio!"

We hospitalized Reed; four days later he was dead.

I was taught in medical school that rheumatic fever "licks the joints, but bites the heart." And so it was with Reed. The acute disease was usually a delayed complication of streptococcal sore throat; it has now been virtually eliminated by treatment of strep infections with penicillin or its antibiotic descendants.

This sad event occurred two generations ago. A few survivors of the earlier polio epidemics are still alive, with permanent loss of muscle function; some suffer from a recurrent polio syndrome. Most people today have no concept of the fear, which at times bordered on hysteria, that gripped parents of young children each summer in the polio era. Reed's mother's reaction was by no means unusual. A few years later the Salk vaccine and then the Sabin vaccine eliminated polio in the United States. Sadly, the job has not been completed—polio has not been eradicated in the world, with persistent pockets in Africa and Asia, despite the availability of the tools to do so. Those of us who cared for patients before the mid-fifties, whether with peripheral muscle involvement or with the bulbar involvement that required the iron lung, will never forget the fear, the horror, and the tragedies.

Dr. White

The Indian Territory created in our area in the 1830s was supposed to remain such forever, but forever is a long time. The Territory became the state of Oklahoma in 1907. One of the "deals" made at the time of entry was that any physician presumably licensed and practicing in the Territory was permitted to practice in the new State without any other requirements or testing. Anyone acquainted with the history of medicine in this country knows that before 1910, many medical schools were proprietary and medical education generally poor, so that the qualifications of physicians prior to that time were suspect. In any case, I heard that somewhere in the nearby hills one of these people, a Dr. White, was still practicing over forty years later. Nobody I knew seemed to know anything about him, other than he was elderly, and nobody in town would have considered going to him. To me, he was only a name of quaint historic interest.

Then, one day, I received a phone call. The caller, a Choctaw man, had been to Dr. White, who had given him a prescription. Both pharmacies in town were apparently closed. Could he have it filled at the Indian Hospital? Technically illegal, I nevertheless agreed, assuming the illness might be serious and the prescription necessary. The man came to the hospital and gave the script to me. The handwriting was shaky, difficult to read, but I was finally able to make it out. Not only did we not have the two medicines written on the prescription, but I had literally never heard of either substance! With regret and an attempt to hide my amazement, I told the man we didn't have those particular medications in stock.

For all I know Dr. White is still practicing somewhere up in those hills!

A Great Success

One afternoon I was called into clinic to see a young Chickasaw man and his son. The father, dressed in dungarees stained with oil, said he had been working on his car engine; his son had been playing nearby.

Suddenly, the father said, the boy started to cough and wheeze. Dad wondered if he had swallowed or breathed in something. The boy, a six-year-old named Clark, was sitting quietly and comfortably while I listened to his father, apparently in no distress. However, when I asked him to hop up on the examining table, he coughed and breathed rapidly for a few seconds. I listened to his chest; intermittently I could hear a rattling sound, like a wheeze, over his central chest when he breathed in and out.

I promptly took him to the x-ray suite and waited impatiently as the technician processed the film. And there it was: some kind of foreign body in the intermediate bronchus—the airway to both the middle and lower lobes of the right lung. It appeared to be a metallic object in the shape of the cap used to connect a spark plug to a car's engine. Not only that, the right lung looked a bit darker than the left. This observation suggested that air could enter the right lung without too much difficulty, but not all of it could be expelled. Apparently air exchange was satisfactory when the boy sat still, but any increased exertion resulted in additional air trapping. This was a dangerous situation. If not immediately treated, it could eventually lead to serious overdistention of the lung with possible rupture and significant pressure on the other lung.

I took the film out to the boys' father; he immediately recognized the metallic cap as such. I pounded on Clark's chest a few times, expecting nothing to happen, and nothing did. I explained the problem. The cap had to be removed, but we did not have the resources at our hospital to do so. The nearest facility with the necessary resources was either in Tulsa or Oklahoma City, both about 200 miles away. I urged the father to keep the boy quiet, but to drive to either hospital immediately. He seemed to agree; he nodded assent, and they left.

The next morning when I came to the hospital I was surprised to see them both sitting on a bench outside the clinic. Clark was much more active than he had been the day before. I greeted them and said, "Boy, that was quick!" I asked what had happened.

"Well, Doc," Dad said, "you know, it's such a long drive to those cities that I decided first to go to the Indian doctor. He looked at the boy, raised up his arms and said some prayers, and the boy coughed and up it came." And he handed me the cap!

It was another lesson for me that there's more than one way to skin a cat, or more things than are dreamt of in my philosophy, or whatever. Even still, I know that, should I be presented with the same situation again, referral to the Indian doctor would not be on my list of options!

A Duck?

"If it looks like a duck, and sounds like a duck, it probably is a duck" is an old medical maxim similar to the one about horses and zebras I stated earlier; both suggest that the common diseases are, indeed, common; while remaining aware of exceptions, one should not look too hard to find them.

Amos, a little five-year-old Creek boy, was brought in, his mother saying he had had the flu for two months, and that I knew his grandpa who had TB, and to whom Amos had been exposed. Amos looked sick. My exam of his right lung was significantly abnormal. The lungs, which are full of air, are usually quite dark on an x-ray, but even his abnormal physical exam did not prepare me for the almost complete "white-out" of Amos's right lung, with a suggestion of a big hole right in its center.

I admitted Amos to the ward with my other child tuberculous patients. His temp was up, and his sputum purulent. However, I could not find the TB germ in it. It was possible his condition might be from a neglected pneumonia, even an abscess, rather than TB, and I treated him for it without much confidence. But penicillin is a marvelous medicine: he improved rapidly, his temp coming down, his appetite returning. And his x-ray cleared as well, leaving him with only some residual thickening of the pleura, the lung lining. It was a pleasant surprise.

The PPD skin test discriminates between individuals who have been infected with the TB germ, whether or not disease is present, and those who have not been exposed and infected. When I first began work in the Indian Bureau I used it often, expecting it to help me in diagnosis. It did not. Almost every single adult and most of the children I saw had a positive test, reflecting the extreme frequency of the infection among Native Americans at that time. Acute illness of almost any cause can

101

depress the body's ability to respond to the test, so I waited until Amos appeared just about completely recovered to test him. His nurses and I watched his little forearm expectantly over the next forty-eight hours, waiting for the usual reaction to appear. To everyone's relief, it did not! Contact with grandpa notwithstanding, Amos had escaped infection— at least so far—and the diagnosis of his illness, a non-tuberculous pneumonia, was confirmed.

So this time the suspected duck—TB—turned out to be some other fowl.

Far enough?

Stella Harjo, a ⅞ Creek woman, was in her early fifties. She had been seen at our hospital a number of times, having had some sort of stroke a few years before. Her blood pressure was high, and she was diabetic; her disease was easily controlled in the hospital, but poorly so at home.

In the spring of 1952 Stella had a new complaint: cough with right-sided chest pain. Her x-ray showed a hazy patch near the base of the right lung; bronchopneumonia was diagnosed and treated with penicillin. She returned in December with similar complaints, her diabetes also out of control. Now, however, her x-ray showed a thin-walled cavity—a hole in the lung—at the site of the previous abnormality. I admitted her.

The diagnostic possibilities included a lung abscess, against which was the lack of a large amount of sputum; cancer, which was very rare in my Indian patients; and tuberculosis. The location in the lower lobe, though unusual for TB, was slightly more common in diabetics. The thin-walled appearance of the cavity suggested and, in fact, was fairly characteristic of a fourth possibility, coccidioidomycosis, colloquially and more easily pronounced as "cocci." This fungus disease is picked up from the soil in the California San Joaquin valley, resulting in what was known as "valley fever" or "desert rheumatism." However, when I asked Stella if she had ever been to California, she said no, claiming she had never been out of Oklahoma.

Despite the lack of sputum I treated her for a lung abscess. Although her TB skin test was positive, I could not recover the TB germ from washings from her stomach into which TB germs are often swallowed. Her x-ray seemed to improve a bit; her clinical condition was stable, and I discharged her to return a few months later.

And return she did, in the spring, with her husband, Alex. Another x-ray showed the cavity in her lung to be smaller, and more thin-walled with no reaction around it, looking even more like cocci. Despite their previous denial of ever being out of Oklahoma, I asked again: have you ever been to California? No. Are you sure? Well, Alex said, not that far. Not that far?! *Where*? The winter prior to her illness they had gone to Florence, Arizona, to pick cotton. Florence! I practically jumped with excitement. Although originally thought to be limited to the San Joaquin valley, cocci was now known to be distributed more widely in the Sonoran life zone. In fact, one of the early evidences of such occurred during World War II. A group of German prisoners of war had been interned in a camp in what was known as the Florence-Eloy-Coolidge triangle in Arizona, and a large group of them had come down with coccidioidomycosis. This was precisely where the Harjo's had picked cotton!

Alex noted my excitement and attention to his wife. I think he became a bit jealous. Well, he said, almost petulantly, I cough too! I took him to the x-ray room, and there it was—he, too, had a cavity, his in the left upper lobe. It was thin-walled, a bit thicker than Stella's, with more reaction around it than expected, but it looked like I had two cases of cocci on my hands! I told them I wanted them both to come into the hospital for more tests. Both couldn't, because of family needs, but Stella could, and when she was ready for discharge, Alex would.

This time in the hospital, I cultured Stella's stomach washings for fungi, and soon saw growth of a white feathery colony on the plate. I then committed a cardinal sin. The form of cocci organism which grows in the lungs and is expectorated is not contagious, that is, the germ is not transmissible from person to person; the infectious form of the fungus is the spore, which persists in the soil, but also develops when the organism is cultured in the laboratory. I packaged up the culture plate and shipped it off to Bethesda for specific identification. The plate broke en route and, when opened in Bethesda, free spores were liberated which could have infected the laboratory workers. Quite properly, I received a letter of admonition, tempered for me by the confirmed identification of the organism as *coccidioides immitis*.

Now that I had established the diagnosis, no treatment was necessary for Stella, as this form of the disease tends to pass off on its own. As agreed, Alex came to the hospital when Stella was discharged. I wonder if you expect the anticlimax. Despite their similar exposure and the relatively similar appearance of the x-ray, Alex's sputum was highly positive—for the TB germ, and his tests for cocci were negative. We started anti-TB treatment, but he could not understand why our attitude about him was so different. After a few months he left the hospital against advice, which he did again after a re-hospitalization a year later. When last seen, his disease was far advanced. I believe he felt the entire situation was unjust, there being no reason why his wife should have received such special treatment!

An aside: cocci is now so common in the Phoenix area that residents there believe the term "valley fever" refers to their valley, not the far distant San Joaquin valley in California.

Family Matters

As I was really a physician caring for a relatively limited population, it is not surprising that I would see more than one member of a family. You have read of Myra Ruth and Etta, mother and daughter, in the Pathologist, and Stella and Alex, husband and wife, above. Later, in the Tuberculosis section, you will read of two other mother-daughter pairs, Emma and Delores, and Virginia and Hinnie Jean. I have one more pair to discuss: Eva Mae and Jamie, brother and sister.

Eva Mae was three years old when I first saw her. A Cherokee of half blood, some of her Caucasian genes were strongly represented in her appearance. She had ringlets of blond hair, a most unusual sight. Her records showed dozens of visits to our clinic, usually for colds or cough. To my surprise, the eventual x-ray showed a pattern of disease in her right upper lung strongly suggestive of the type of tuberculosis commonly seen in adults rather than children. The sputum we recovered did show the TB germ, and I began standard treatment; she did well. A second surprise occurred in her contact evaluations, that is, in trying to determine who might have exposed her to the disease. In adults, the source from whom a person probably contracted the disease is often difficult to find. In children, however, the reverse is true, since their contacts are often limited to the family or others close to the family. That is how I met Eva Mae's parents and brother, Jamie, five years older than Eva Mae, all of whom had no evidence of tuberculosis. Eva Mae was hospitalized for just a few months, a relatively short time for the era, and I saw her with her family again in two follow-up visits. Everyone was pleased with the positive outcome.

On the third visit the mother asked me to look at Jamie. She was concerned, because he too was coughing and, she said, seemed to have trouble breathing at night. When I examined him, I did, indeed, hear some noisy breath sounds; in addition, his face and neck seemed swollen, and I could feel some enlarged lymph nodes on the left. I took a chest x-ray and was both surprised and appalled at what I discovered. Jamie had a gigantic mass of abnormal tissue filling the mediastinum, the space between the two lungs. I recalled that his records shortly after birth showed Jamie had received radiation therapy for an enlarged thymus gland in a nearby city. Now on biopsy a lymph node was replaced by lymphoma appearing cells, his disease perhaps a late complication of the radiation he had received as an infant. Radiation therapy was begun, but his white blood cell count, at first normal, soon markedly increased, and these cells were abnormal. Jamie had either some form of a lymphoma which had spilled over into his blood stream, or a leukemia with marked tissue invasion.

The family was told the prognosis was very poor. Radiation was discontinued. I told them recent advances in the treatment of leukemia and this sort of tumor held out some hope; they would have to take Jamie to a major medical center—there was one in Oklahoma City—and I recommended they do so.

105

This was at a time prior to medical insurance, in the days when poor people often had to depend on the charity of major institutions. Our discussion was somber. I could see they were torn between naturally wanting to do whatever they could for their son, and the hard reality of his prognosis, given the massive economic burden it presented. They left. The mood of this family visit was horribly different from our previous experiences together.

I heard a few weeks later that Jamie had died at home.

An Improved Position

Our medical center, the Indian Hospital, was a major employer in Talihina. The other was the state tuberculosis sanatorium of eastern Oklahoma, not far away on an adjacent hill. I appreciated its close proximity and utilized the expertise of the physicians there. Dr. Baker, the director, and his staff were all experienced phthisiologists—tuberculosis physicians—especially in surgical techniques. They were slow, however, to embrace the emerging practice of chemotherapy and were disdainful of me, a young whippersnapper, for favoring this new kind of drug therapy. I believe that, while they respected my ability, they were reluctant to show it openly. But then came Bucky Rollins.

I had toured their sanatorium, and they had shown me some of their cases. During my second year in Talihina, I was surprised when Dr. Baker asked me for help with a patient, one Bucky Rollins. Rollins had tested negative for TB, and his condition puzzled Baker. Dr. Baker first showed me the x-ray, which was markedly abnormal. The right side showed multiple feathery densities throughout the right lung, fanning out from its central root. Heavier centrally and above, but involving the entire lung, the shadows obscured the outlines of the normal blood vessels. The appearance strongly suggested pulmonary congestion and edema to me, such as one would see with heart failure, and the heart even seemed a bit enlarged. But the left lung was entirely clear! Heart failure should have involved both lungs symmetrically. It was hard to think of a reason, or condition, for the asymmetrical appearance. I probed for further information about Rollins. Baker said he was a local middle-aged farmer, who complained of cough and shortness of breath. He was rather vague about the physical findings. As fluid collections and congestion can be affected by gravity, I asked about Rollins' position in bed—did he prefer, for some reason, to lie only on his right side? Baker and his staff didn't know.

We went over to their hospital for me to examine the man. When I entered his room, there he was, half propped up, lying on his right side. And when I took off his blanket and bed covering, there it was: his left leg had been amputated just below the hip. The stump, and the right foot, were swollen. It was uncomfortable for him to lie on the amputated side, and he naturally spent his time on the right. I prescribed the fairly simple heart failure therapy available then; it resulted in considerable fluid loss by diuresis. The foot edema and the unilateral congestion also cleared.

It turned out that Baker and his staff were aware of the amputation, the result of a gun shot accident while hunting, not uncommon in our area. But they had not put two and two together. I encouraged Rollins to change his position frequently while in bed; his condition and my reputation—and position—all improved considerably!

Susie Bright Eyes

I will always think of her as Susie Bright Eyes. For a twelve-year-old, her appearance was stunning: tall for her age, braided hair, freckles—so unusual they immediately identified her as not of full Indian blood—and a shining brightness in her eyes. Her fever probably accentuated the brightness, but when she spoke and responded to questions, those eyes shone with intelligence, humor, and a brightness of spirit.

She had had severe abdominal pain a week or so previously, pain that caused her to cry, to stay home from school, to lose sleep. Her mother said it was probably indigestion. Some home medicines seemed to help, and a day or two later the pain subsided. She didn't feel better, however, and her fever, which had been mild at first, increased. She had vomited a few times. Finally into clinic they came.

Her temp was over 103, her skin hot and dry, her abdomen firm and tense. We agreed on the diagnosis: acute appendicitis. Neglected, the appendix had ruptured, and she now had diffuse peritonitis. Along with my two colleagues—Dr. Roberts and Dr. Cooper, I'll call them—I took her directly to the operating room.

Roberts, as always, was the surgeon. Reversing roles with Cooper, I assisted Roberts, and Cooper gave the anesthesia. We used ether, dripped onto a cone shaped mask. Before Cooper began the anesthesia, Susie smiled and made a cheerful remark. Try as I may, I cannot remember the words; but I can still see the smile.

Roberts's incision was small; when he entered the abdomen he sucked free pus from the abdominal cavity. He easily found the appendix, angrily inflamed, swollen and ruptured. He removed it. Long before the days of monitors in the operating room, as he began to cauterize the base of the appendix, I noticed that the blood oozing from her wounds was dark, maroon, rather than the expected bright red. Cooper couldn't find a pulse—her heart had stopped beating. Today we would immediately recognize this as a cardiac arrest and would apply CPR, but this was 1952 before external cardiac resuscitation had been described. But open cardiac massage had been reported, and I encouraged a reluctant Roberts to open the chest and do so. He did and, fortunately, Susie's heart started beating again. Roberts quickly closed the abdominal and chest incisions. But Susie had stopped breathing on her own. We supplied oxygen, and squeezed an air containing bag positioned over her face; we were gratified to see her blood pink up. Each time we removed the bag, however, she did not resume spontaneous breathing on her own.

So, there we were. What had happened? I realized I, the internist, had erred in not stopping to think before agreeing to take her directly to the operating room. Her appendix had already ruptured; we should have started antibiotics, brought down her fever and improved her hydration before subjecting her to surgery and anesthesia—the cardiac arrest was the result of the additional strain. Then, during the period of lack of heart beat, it appeared that her brain had been damaged in the area responsible for spontaneous breathing. It was analogous to the bulbar form of polio, still common in those days, which affected that part of the brain. Bulbar polio was treated by putting the patient in an iron lung until, hopefully, spontaneous breathing returned. I did not think about the rest of her brain: the concept of "brain death" was still in the future, and I hoped and assumed with time she would awaken.

We took Susie from the operating room and connected her to a intermittent positive pressure breathing machine, which regularly expanded her lungs. After a few trials it became clear she needed both oxygen and the artificial ventilation to keep her heart pumping and her color pink.

We were surely not equipped to handle the situation. I knew there was a polio unit in Tulsa, almost 200 miles away. I called, and after being shifted from one person to another with much discussion and argument, I finally received a reluctant agreement to admit her there.

But how to get her to Tulsa? Helicopters were not yet a possibility. We had no ambulance. The undertaker in town, my friend David Drake, did have a big hearse. I called, and he was willing to help. We managed to get an oxygen tank into the hearse, and Susie on a stretcher alongside it. It took trial, error and tubing to connect her up to the various machines. Finally, late at night, we started out: David, driving, along with me and Miss Van Beekum, a resourceful and competent nurse. David drove carefully along the unlit two lane roads, over the mountains, wending us north towards Tulsa. The family followed in their old beat up pickup truck.

Soon, too soon, the battery supplying our ventilating machine failed, and Susie's pulse slowed. After a flurry of excitement, she improved as we manually, rhythmically, squeezed the ventilating bag. Miss Van and I spelled each other. David drove on in the dark night. And then, suddenly, around 2 a.m., the plastic suction tubing we had used as a connection from the oxygen tank to Susie blew up like a balloon and burst. We had no replacement. I stood outside the hearse, smoking, looking up at the starry sky, searching for a solution, conferring with the others. There was nothing we could do. And so, on a lonely road in the middle of the night, Susie's bright eyes were extinguished forever.

Tuberculosis

Spes phthisica

Have you seen "La Traviata"? It is a lovely opera by Giuseppe Verdi. In it the heroine, Violetta, has tuberculosis, as do many operatic heroines. In fact, one wag claimed that were it not for TB, romantic opera of the 19th century would not have survived. In any case, the final act of "La Traviata" opens with Violetta on her death bed, weak, frail, terminally ill. She is reunited with her lover, but their hopes are dashed as she falls back to bed, exhausted. Then, just before the final curtain, she rises and lustily sings: "The pain is gone. I feel life returning. Oh, Joy!!!" She then falls dead as the curtain descends.

That final scene is beautiful, touching even, but, I used to think, really silly. I was convinced this optimism in the face of death was simply a theatrical contrivance. Then I met Henry Mathews. I was a third year medical student on the wards of Cook County Hospital. Mr. Mathews, an elderly black man, lay in one of the beds in the center of the ward, covers pulled up to his grizzled chin. He had disseminated tuberculosis, primarily manifesting itself as tuberculous peritonitis (infection of the internal lining of the abdomen). Indeed, when I examined him I found his abdomen swollen, tense and tender, the skin warm to the touch. I asked him how he felt. He smiled and said, "Jes' fine, doc." And so it was each morning as I came onto the ward.

At his bedside I asked, "How are you today, Henry?" The response, with a smile, was always the same—jes' fine.

Then one morning Mathews was not there. His bed was empty and freshly made.

Later that day I attended Mathews's autopsy. The glistening lining of his peritoneal cavity was studded with millions of tiny spots, each a "tubercle"—a tiny focus which contained the TB germ, plus the tissue reaction to it. Not only the peritoneum was involved; the spots, called miliary tubercles after their resemblance to tiny bird seeds, were uniform through his organs. Yet he, while alive, had remained cheerful and uncomplaining.

I later learned that this generally optimistic and cheerful outlook of the seriously ill tuberculous patient was a well-known and long-recognized phenomenon. It had an ancient name: spes phthisica, variously translated to reflect the hopeful attitude of the tuberculous patient. The commonest definition, perhaps, is a state of euphoria occurring in patients with tuberculosis. Other commentators, impressed with the long list of artists, poets and musicians who died young following remarkable outbursts of creative energy, postulated that the physical wasting of these patients had led to a euphoric flowering of the passionate and creative aspects of the soul. Mr. Mathews did, indeed, exhibit such optimism and cheerfulness; I cannot speak to the flowering of Mr. Mathews's soul.

In later years I would again be impressed with similar behavior among many of my patients. I recall one young Navajo boy, who sketched a caricature of me as a present the day before he died. In any case, I no longer consider Violetta's positive outlook in the face of death to be a silly, over-theatrical contrivance; rather, it is as moving and poignant as that which can occur in real life.

Background

Tuberculosis is primarily a disease of the lungs. Pulmonary tuberculosis was a major killer throughout the world for centuries. The tuberculosis germ destroys areas of the lung creating holes, termed cavities; within them, the germs grow apace. The organisms are then able easily to spread elsewhere in the lungs. Major, sometimes fatal, hemorrhages can arise from the cavities. The dangerous organisms can also be expectorated and potentially infect others. A major goal of treatment was, therefore, to close these cavities. If this could be accomplished, general healing might ensue; if it could not, the patient's course was usually progressive and, most likely, fatal.

From the late 19th century onward methods of treatment for tuberculosis, though well established, had limited success. The keynote was sanatorium care, which isolated the patient from his contacts and hopefully protected society from the spread of this contagious disease. For the patient, sanatorium care included strict bed rest, fresh air, a healthy diet, and removal from the physical and emotional stresses of everyday life, plus the availability of physicians knowledgeable about the disease and skilled in additional treatment methods. If bed rest was inadequate to close the cavities, mechanical collapse procedures could be instituted. These collapse methods gradually gave way to surgical methods involving the actual removal of diseased portions of the lungs. We learned later that even this approach was unnecessary.

The 1940s saw the development of the antibiotic streptomycin, which could potentially halt the progression of the more virulent forms of tuberculosis. It was rarely curative. It wasn't until the arrival of isoniazid in 1952 that the real conquest of tuberculosis began. Isoniazid eventually permitted the closure of the sanatoria and led to the modern approach to treatment, which involves multiple anti-tuberculous agents, administered to outpatients for at least six months, preferably under the direct supervision of health care personnel. This approach results in control and cure of the disease with a remarkably small relapse rate for patients whose germs remain susceptible to chemotherapy. Note that, although today the term "chemotherapy" often refers to the treatment of tumors, it actually means treatment with chemical substances. It is a term I prefer when referring to tuberculosis treatment, since not all the agents we use in tuberculosis therapy are antibiotics.

It was my good fortune to start my career in tuberculosis during the transition from the pre-chemotherapy era ("collapse" and surgical procedures) to the present one of curative chemotherapy. Many of my already hospitalized Indian Bureau patients had received each new agent as it became available; their germs had severally developed resistance to each; they thus resembled patients in the pre-chemotherapy era. I was also involved, with new patients, in the development of understanding how these agents were to be most efficiently utilized.

It was an exciting time to be working in the field of tuberculosis. I was quite busy. We averaged fifteen admissions per month to the sanatorium, with the same average number of discharges. Unfortunately, only a minority of these were discharged alive and well, with permission.

Tuberculosis was, and is, a fascinating disorder, with a long, even romantic, history. I learned much about the natural history and treatment of the disease, but also, as these stories will reveal, the interrelationships between the germ, the people who suffered with it, and society.

In Training

In medical school we had, of course, been taught in formal classes about tuberculosis, and I understood it as a common chronic and deadly illness of the lungs. Most of my clerkships—my clinical training—were at the Cook County Hospital. One morning we were called to the morgue to witness an autopsy. We saw a twelve-year-old boy stretched out on the table. We were told the history: the boy had been ill for only ten days, with fever and headache, and had declined rapidly. The autopsy showed a thick exudate (collection of inflammatory fluid) covering the lining of the brain, particularly at its base. The diagnosis was tuberculous meningitis. I was struck by the rapidity with which the illness led to death, and by its presence elsewhere than in the lungs. There was clearly more to this deadly disease than I first realized.

Dr. Amberson

One person, a teacher of mine, stands out in my memory. He taught me and countless others much about tuberculosis, about medicine, and about the relationship of physicians to patients and colleagues.

J. Burns Amberson, MD, was Professor of Medicine at Columbia University Medical School. He was also head of the Chest Service at Bellevue Hospital in New York City, arguably the outstanding program for the training of pulmonary and tuberculosis physicians in the years before and after World War II. He was a formal, quiet, conservative man of immense knowledge and experience. He was one of the founders of the discipline of pulmonary medicine, broadening it beyond tuberculosis alone. When he spoke, everyone listened; his statements were authoritative. To my good luck, he was also a consultant in pulmonary disease at the Bronx VA during the years I trained there. I was thus a house officer when I had my first contact with him.

Dr. Amberson came to our hospital on Saturday mornings for presentation of cases to him by the residents. One morning, Dr. Frank Lovelock, chief of our service, selected a patient whose disease was undiagnosed. Still in training, my appreciation of the x-ray appearance was not sophisticated. I recall, probably incorrectly, that it showed two round nodules in each lung, a smaller one above, a larger below. Dr. Amberson studied the films and said, "Well, I don't know what this is, but one thing I feel certain about, it is not tuberculosis." A few weeks later the cultures of the sputum returned positive for the tuberculosis germ. Dr. Lovelock decided to present the patient to Dr. Amberson again the next Saturday, without divulging the new information. Once again, Dr. Amberson studied the x-rays. "Well," he said, "I don't know what this is, but I think the most likely diagnosis is tuberculosis."

"But Dr. Amberson," we remonstrated, "a few weeks ago tuberculosis was the one diagnosis you thought this was not!"

"Well," said Dr. Amberson, "if you say that is what I said, I am sure I did. But today I cannot see how I could have done so!"

I remember being very impressed. I learned one can evaluate the same evidence quite differently at different times with no clear knowledge of why. I learned also that diagnosis is not only difficult, but that findings and the reasoning associated with those findings are not hard and fast. Most importantly, I learned the humility of accepting one's own mistakes and fallibility, as well as being open to other points of view. These valuable points have remained with me, although I am certain I have at times failed to heed them.

This was but one example of a lesson from Dr. Amberson; we remained in contact for many years. He was surely a role model to be admired.

Charlie Vandenbosch

Perhaps the most instructive patient I had as a medical resident was Charlie Vandenbosch. I had seen rheumatoid arthritis before, both in its chronic and acute forms. I particularly remember a young housewife in her twenties with exquisitely swollen and tender joints. But until Charles Vandenbosch, I had never been responsible for the care of someone with a long-term history of the disease, chronic disability, AND an acute flare-up. Probably for the first time I made an extensive drawing in the chart, noting the swelling, the pain, the deformity, the involvement of each and every joint.

Charlie became quite attached to me; in fact, he became dependent. A man in his forties, he had no family that I remember. He may have been gay, something we rarely considered at the time.

I tried all the usual treatment options of the day, such as they were—aspirin and multiple physical methods. We used a long course of injected gold, but that too was ineffective. It is not an exaggeration to say Charlie was in considerable pain. Finally, after much discussion and consultation, it was agreed that Charles was a good candidate for a fairly new form of treatment: adrenal steroids—cortisone. Anyone reading this some fifty years later may find it surprising that this decision required discussion. Although known to be powerful and effective in treating rheumatoid arthritis, steroids were new and expensive; and the complications associated with steroid treatment were still being learned.

116

Nonetheless, it was decided that Charles's new treatment would begin the following Monday.

Charles's chest x-ray had been normal on admission; in hindsight I am not certain of my motivation for what I did next. Perhaps it was as simple as being part of standard protocol; perhaps it was a lucky move; or perhaps it was because I somehow knew that steroids could exacerbate tuberculosis. Whatever the reason, I ordered a chest x-ray to be taken on Friday as a baseline before starting the steroid treatment. Lo and behold, his x-ray showed the presence of fairly advanced TB, involving a good bit of the right upper lobe. Poor Charles! He was transferred to the Tuberculosis ward where, incidentally, I later again took care of him, but his steroid therapy was canceled and anti-TB treatment begun instead. He continued to suffer, and it was not until many months later when the TB was under control that we were willing, nervously and cautiously, to begin cortisone treatment. His response was moderate, but gratifying.

The lesson here is a simple, but important one: if you are going to make a basic change in treatment, or in its direction, make sure you mark each change with a chest x-ray (or with repeat basic data—for example, liver function tests in that circumstance). I have seen (and still see!) instances in which a patient is diagnosed with tuberculosis (or pneumonia, or cancer, or whatever); work up takes a week or more; treatment is begun; on a repeat x-ray shortly thereafter, the condition is worse. The conclusion often is that the treatment is ineffective; but an x-ray just before treatment might well have shown progression before the treatment was started. And, in fact, the new x-ray may actually be improved, but there is no way to know unless an x-ray on the day of change was done. And, when I think of this important principle, it is Charles Vanderbosch who always comes to mind.

Compliance

Sanatorium life was not easy for most people. In addition to the obvious distress of being separated from family and friends and from normal surroundings, many found the key aspect of treatment, enforced bed rest, difficult. The sexual deprivation was especially trying for many young people. Also, the length of hospitalization, measured not in days or months, but often in years, was a requirement many could not tolerate. It was common to hear rationalizations such as "you are only treating me with bed rest; I could do that at home;" or, "you are only treating me with pneumothorax (administered once a week); I can go home and come back for that;" or later, "you are only treating me with medicines; I could take them at home." There was truth in each of these rationalizations, but we did not know it at the time. It wasn't until years later when we had adequate experience with chemotherapy, plus epidemiologic evidence, that we could confirm these options. Today initial periods of hospitalization are often required for sick people with tuberculosis, but the bulk of treatment consists of taking medications which, is, indeed, carried out at home, often under direct supervision.

Emmaline

Emmaline James was, literally, a beautiful girl—not just pretty or pleasant looking, but beautiful. She had big eyelashes, dark eyes, and a mole on her cheek that demonstrated why moles were called beauty spots. She was a Choctaw of ¾ blood, and that other quarter must have been strong, because she had a pale-skinned olive complexion that added to her beauty.

She had entered the sanatorium before I arrived at Talihina, just before her fifteenth birthday, with recent symptoms of lethargy, cough and chest pain. She had a big left pleural effusion (a collection of fluid due to tuberculous inflammation) in the space between the lungs and the rib cage. The fluid was "tapped," that is, partially removed. She was put to bed and given three weeks of daily streptomycin. The effusion cleared, and she improved clinically. Gradually she returned to full activity. Shortly after I arrived, when she had been in the hospital almost a year, and just before her contemplated discharge, her x-ray now showed new disease in the left upper lobe of her lung, and the tuberculosis germ was grown from washings of swallowed phlegm collected from her stomach. This recrudescence was unexpected and disappointing, but not surprising. Many patients developed tuberculosis in the lungs within a year or two of a pleural effusion; we now know the treatment she had been given was neither adequate nor particularly effective. I restricted her activity and put her on streptomycin and the oral medication PAS, but she lost weight and seemed listless, probably due to the unexpected relapse.

Emmaline somehow reminded me of the Jean Simmons character in one episode of the film "Trio," adapted from the Somerset Maugham story "Sanatorium." In the movie Michael Rennie plays a roué who has come to the sanatorium and, to his surprise, falls in love with Simmons. His disease is chronic, with a current relapse from which he is expected to recover; her disease is such that she can only survive under the protected conditions of sanatorium life, as it is likely to progress and even cause death, if subjected to the strains of normal living. When they speak to the sanatorium physician about their desire to marry and leave the san, he tells them that, although Rennie probably still has some few years to live, she is unlikely to survive for more than six months. In full realization of what it means, they, nevertheless, decide to leave the sanatorium together. It was Emmaline's beauty and similar condition that reminded me of the romantic Jean Simmons character.

After a few months on the new regimen Emmaline's x-ray improved, although she did not change much clinically. Her parents took her from the sanatorium against my advice in the fall. I saw her on the street in Talihina the next summer. She was sixteen, pale, thin and beautiful.

About a year after we returned to New York, I heard that Emmaline had been readmitted with far advanced tuberculosis. She died before her 20th birthday.

The Youthful Imperative

In the 19th century the Choctaw Indians had been moved from Mississippi to Indian Territory, which later became Oklahoma. A band of Choctaws had remained in Mississippi, and Pearl Lee Vancil was descended from them. A pretty girl of nineteen, she had been coughing and losing weight for some months before her tuberculosis was diagnosed. She was transferred and hospitalized in the sanatorium in Talihina. Sadly, her x-ray showed extensive disease involving most of the left lung, with spread to the right as well. Her response to treatment was slow and not continuous, and her sputum persistently revealed the TB germ. It was clear her condition was fragile, and her ability to resist the disease, tenuous. Gradually, however, she began to improve, especially after isoniazid became available. As commonly occurs, improvement in her sense of well-being long preceded actual improvement in the status of her disease. After eighteen months of hospitalization, it began to look as if left-sided thoracoplasty, a deforming surgical procedure, might control her disease.

Burt Waller's illness presented a different scenario. Also a Mississippi Choctaw, now twenty-eight, his tuberculosis had been originally diagnosed ten years earlier, when he was eighteen. He had had at least four prior hospitalizations at another Indian Bureau sanatorium in Shawnee, Oklahoma. Each hospitalization had been caused by an increase in his symptoms; at each hospitalization, with bed rest and occasional chemotherapy, his symptoms had been controlled. From each of these he had absconded, leaving against medical advice with his disease still active. His course was typical of someone for whom the phrase "good chronic" was invented. It described a patient with chronic disease who, nevertheless, seemed to have good resistance. Major progression to serious or fatal illness did not occur. Many of us resisted use of the term, as there was nothing really "good" about this situation— the patient's sputum usually remained positive, and they undoubtedly continued to spread the disease to others.

Long-term hospitalization is very difficult for anyone, but especially so for young people who are feeling relatively well. To counter their isolation, I instituted a program in the sanatorium in which, on Wednesday afternoons, we held a social gathering for those patients whose conditions permitted a certain level of activity. We supplied cards and other games, snacks and soft drinks. We played music on the radio and, sometimes, records, although we did not permit dancing. The men and women usually sat at tables and talked. They eagerly looked forward to these weekly sessions. Indeed, I became a "special delivery" mail man—on rounds I was often given a note to be delivered to a patient of the opposite sex. I noticed that Pearl Lee and Burt were exchanging messages frequently. And then, one morning on rounds, I found they were both gone. One of the other patients told me that during the night a pickup truck had pulled up to one of the back windows of the sanatorium, and Pearl Lee and Burt had left together. I never heard from them again. While I was disappointed and felt I had failed by not impressing upon them the need to remain hospitalized, in my heart I wished the young couple well.

Although it was Emmaline who had first reminded me of "Trio," it felt as if I was watching the romantic story play out with Pearl Lee and Burt's escape. As with the couple in the movie, they had apparently decided to leave the sanatorium and grasp some happiness from life.

Mary Martha

While I was in the Indian Bureau I never adequately realized the background romance of some of my patients' names. The surname of one of them, for example, was "Ameahtubbee," which has a classic Chickasaw ending. And "Leflore" was the name of another patient, of a Choctaw hero, of a county in Mississippi, and of our adjacent county in Talihina.

Mary Martha Leflore, ¾ Choctaw, was first seen at our hospital at age seventeen when, after a sore throat, she had ankle swelling and headache. A year later, pregnant, she was seen twice, first for threatened premature birth, and then again when she was hospitalized for her expected delivery. Because of the high prevalence of tuberculosis in the population our hospital served, my policy was to take a chest x-ray on everyone admitted. Thus on that admission in November 1952, Mary Martha had a chest x-ray. It was abnormal, with a minimal infiltrate in each upper lobe. I told her she had TB and needed to be treated, but I was unable to convince her she had the disease, as she had no symptoms. Mary Martha left against advice, the baby undelivered, and she gave birth shortly thereafter at home. The next spring she was seen twice with chest pain, fever, and recurrent "colds." Her x-ray now showed a cavity in the left upper lung with spread inferiorly in that lung—and asymmetric breasts, as she was nursing the infant. Again, she refused hospitalization. When finally admitted in June 1954, a year and a half after the first diagnosis, her weight had gone from 137 to 90 pounds; her disease was now bilateral and far advanced. Her positive sputum proved she had TB. She improved on treatment, but left the hospital against advice after six weeks. After I had returned to New York I learned she had a similar short admission the next year, but had died in 1956 at age twenty-two. The nursing staff said she was just unable to adjust to sanatorium life.

Mary Martha illustrates not only the natural, inexorable course of untreated tuberculosis in susceptible patients, but also the issue of doctor failure versus patient noncompliance. I considered my failure to convince her to stay my shortcoming as a physician; given the same situation today, the patient would be labeled "noncompliant." It is too easy for physicians today to assign patient's unwillingness to follow their recommendations to "noncompliance;" in my mind, the responsibility should be shared mutually.

Perseverance

I must contrast the prior three examples of "noncompliance" with the remarkable story of medical care and patient perseverance exemplified by Bette Sue.

A full blooded Choctaw, Bette Sue was seventeen when first admitted in April 1949. She had been ill with fever, cough and hoarseness for only three weeks, but her x-ray showed cavitary tuberculous disease in the left upper lobe, with similar changes, yet without a definite cavity, on the right. Her sputum was heavily positive for the TB germ (and was to remain so for five years!). Artificial pneumothorax (air put into the chest between the chest wall lining and the lung to collapse the diseased portions of lung) was attempted, but was unsuccessful. A short period of pneumoperitoneum—air placed into the abdomen to provide upward pressure on the lungs—was given. Streptomycin had recently been described as effective in tuberculosis, but at first the Indian Bureau apparently did not have funds to stock it. Ten grams of streptomycin was purchased by her family for $100 and 0.5 gram given daily by injection; it was then continued intermittently throughout that year for a total of 90 gm. At first Bette Sue seemed to improve, with clearing in her right lung, but by the end of the year, her disease involved most of the left lung.

In 1950 an oral drug, (para)aminosalicylic acid (PAS), became available. Each pill weighed 0.5 gm, the daily dose was 12 gm, which meant twenty-four pills per day. She was given it, sometimes with the streptomycin, sometimes alone. PAS was an unpleasant medication to take, upsetting the GI tract. (Later, in the days of outpatient treatment, it was said that a three-month supply of isoniazid lasted three months, while a three-month supply of PAS lasted indefinitely.) Bette Sue also received another oral drug, amithiozone (its clever trade name was "tibione," or "TB One"). TB One was popular in Europe, but never in favor in the US. Again, to no avail; by the end of 1950 Bette Sue's left lung was essentially destroyed. Her hoarseness was due to TB of the larynx.

In 1951 her disease spread to the right. Despite this being her only functioning lung, artificial pneumothorax was instituted and kept up for six months. The right-sided disease cleared. A bothersome rash, common in sanatorium patients, had also appeared, primarily affecting her hands.

I arrived in 1952 after she had been in the sanatorium for three years. Streptomycin and PAS, to which her germs were now undoubtedly resistant, were being administered only intermittently. Her clinical condition was fair and her weight stable, despite a destroyed left lung, positive sputum, chronic cough, hoarseness and rash. Isoniazid (INH), the wonder drug, was also now available, but I realized two things: first, were she ever to be "cured," she would require removal of the entire left lung; second, that I would surely need INH to protect her at the time of surgery, and were I to give her that single drug now, her TB organisms would likely become resistant to it too. The surgery would be extremely difficult and complicated, far beyond our capabilities at Talihina. I began to work on arrangements with another Indian Bureau sanatorium, in Shawnee OK, near Oklahoma City, where complex surgery could be done.

Then in April 1953, after increased cough with some expectoration of blood, the disease again spread to the right lower lung. My hands were tied. I started the isoniazid and, somewhat later, also instituted pneumoperitoneum to compress that now diseased lower lung. Success! Not only did the right lung disease clear and stabilize, the hoarseness resolved, and the rash cleared as well! It may have been lupus vulgaris, tuberculosis of the skin, or a peculiar skin reaction, called a tuberculid, occasionally seen in sanatorium patients.

It is now 1954. And what of Bette Sue, the person, the human being, the woman, to whom all this was happening? She was fair-skinned, pretty by any standards, intelligent, and uniformly cheerful and optimistic. Our conversations during the regular reviews of her status were always warm and friendly. In bed for most days all those years with only a few visitors, her social contacts (as far as I knew) were limited to the once-a-week social gatherings we had created for the men and women, and the occasional holiday party. In that era patients left the sanatorium against advice much too frequently, but to my knowledge, Bette Sue never left and never complained, all the while growing from an awkward teenager into an attractive young woman.

Finally, early in 1954, Bette Sue was transferred to Shawnee for the operation. An extrapleural pneumonectomy was performed—as the space between the lung and the chest wall had been entirely destroyed, the dissection had to be carried out just under the ribs in the chest wall itself. The procedure was successful. After the postoperative period Bette Sue returned to Talihina. Her x-ray appeared unchanged—the destroyed airless left lung had now been replaced by blood and fluid filling the vacant space which cast a similar shadow. (In fact, I used her x-rays to teach what I termed the Resh sign, the subtle change in the sweep of the ribs, now interrupted by a surgical defect.) I continued her pneumoperitoneum for a while, and then discontinued it. For the first time in almost six years her sputum was negative for TB bacilli, and she was no longer in danger of hemorrhage or spread.

I returned to New York that September. By plan, all chemotherapy for Bette Sue was discontinued, and she went home over Christmas for the first time since she had been admitted. She was discharged shortly thereafter, in 1955, at age twenty-three. She had been in the sanatorium six years, the same time period that an inteflex student at Michigan could go from high school to the MD degree.

Some years later I received a life insurance form from her to fill out. She was living in Knoxville, Tennessee. I was absolutely delighted to know she was alive and apparently doing well. I lost track of her after that.

Bette Sue is a study in human perseverance and courage, in striking contrast to the noncompliant many. I hope she is as proud of herself as I am of her. Her story is not unique, yet it does not detract one iota from its remarkableness.

Standard Approaches to Treatment
Emma—and Delores

Emma Vann was a healthy forty-two-year-old Cherokee woman. Her husband was an attendant at the hospital, and they had a good standard of living. One morning while shopping in town, Emma felt what she described as a scratchy feeling in her chest; she cleared her throat, spat into a tissue, and was shocked to see a glob of bright red blood. That very day she reported to the hospital. An x-ray was taken. There, in the left upper lobe, was the cause of the blood spitting. A thick-walled hole in the lung, a cavity, was easily discerned. The tissue above it was thickened, while around it a few additional hazy spots suggested spread of the disease. I hospitalized her immediately.

Emma had had absolutely no other symptoms; nevertheless, the diagnosis of tuberculosis was obvious and was confirmed by the presence of innumerable TB germs in a stained smear of her sputum. I ordered her to bed, left side down, with an ice pack on her chest. The next day the bloody expectoration—hemoptysis—recurred; more blood, a few tablespoons, this time. Emma was at risk for a major life-threatening hemorrhage; in addition, it was well known that hemoptysis in tuberculosis created fertile ground for spread of disease to other portions of the lungs.

For the more than a half century before the days of the modern antituberculosis drugs, the first question phthisologists (tuberculosis physicians) asked themselves when new patients were admitted to the sanatorium was "Is the situation appropriate for artificial pnemothorax?" If the answer was yes, this procedure was often employed in routine and emergency situations. In artificial pneumothorax, air (or some other gas) was introduced into the pleural space, a potential space between the overlying ribs and underlying lung. The elastic lung would then "collapse," and the degree of collapse could be controlled. Fortunately, experience had taught that diseased portions of the lung tended to collapse more than normal lung; thus, a cavity might well be closed, reducing the risk of further hemorrhage and additional spread. The procedure was not always successful; it was never subjected to the sort of randomized trials one would require for scientific evidence today, but those of us who used it were convinced it saved many, many lives.

Initial pneumothorax was technically a somewhat difficult procedure. I had an apparatus, the Davidson pneumothorax device, which permitted me to control the amount of air injected. Fortunately, the pressure within the pleural space is negative, that is, less than atmospheric; when the tip of my exploring needle entered the potential space, anaesthetizing fluid in the barrel of my syringe was sucked in. I then could switch to the Davidson and let air enter. And this I did the next morning for Emma. The procedure went well; she had no negative symptoms or resultant shortness of breath. I repeated the procedure every day for the next few days, and then expectantly took a new x-ray. To my dismay, I found that the normal lower lobe of the lung had collapsed, but the thick tissue superior to the cavity, representing broad fibrous bands, had attached the lung to the pleural lining on the interior of the chest wall, and these bands were still holding the cavity open.

Fortunately, an additional procedure was available. The surgeon at the nearby state tuberculosis sanatorium was adept at a procedure termed "pneumonolysis"—freeing of the lung. A lighted scope was introduced into the air-filled pleural space through the chest wall, accompanied by a cauterizing instrument. The adhesions—the fibrous bands—were visualized and then zapped by the cautery. This procedure was successful for Emma; the lung fell away from the chest wall.

A note about the management of pneumothorax: before each scheduled refill of air, I would fluoroscope the patient, assess the degree of collapse, and determine how much air I would introduce at the refill. As I had many patients receiving pneumothorax, as well as an analogous procedure in the abdomen, pneumoperitoneum, I would fluoroscope them one after the other. Today technological improvements permit fluoroscopy—still a common technique for colonoscopy and other gastrointestinal procedures, for example—to be done in a well-lighted room. Not so then. The room had to be totally dark, since the fluoroscopic screen glowed only faintly. In fact, it was first necessary to accommodate one's eyes for night vision to see accurately. The options were to spend a half hour or so sitting in the dark, doing nothing else, or to wear red goggles in advance for the same length of time, thus permitting one's eyes to accommodate while performing other activities. One of the extremely skilled men who taught me fluoroscopy, Dr. John Schwedel, actually wore dark sun glasses all day long to remain accommodated at a time long before such glasses were fashionable. His appearance, walking down the halls of the hospital, was quite unusual for those days, to say the least.

Back to Emma. When her fluoroscopy and x-rays were repeated, the upper lung was shown to have collapsed as well; the cavity was compressed and partially closed. Emma was out of immediate danger.

Meanwhile, we called in Emma's family contacts to check them for disease. The x-rays of her husband Bentley, her son Bradley and her fif-teen-year-old daughter, Delores, were all normal. But Delores's x-ray had an interesting feature. At the root of the left lung, I could see clear-cut calcifications in the lymph nodes. I assumed these were evidence of prior tuberculous infection. At that time I did not realize they also could be residua of infection with the soil fungus *Histoplasma capsulatum*. Studies demonstrating the ubiquitousness of this fungus had not yet been done.

Emma did well; I treated her with pneumothorax "refills" weekly, fluoroscoping her before each session to ascertain the degree of lung collapse, and then giving what I thought should be the appropriate volume of air. The hemoptysis did not recur; after two months her sputum became negative. As she lived in town, and was clearly a reliable patient, I discharged her to home. Our plan was to continue the pneumothorax treatments for at least a year, perhaps two, to assure healing of the tuberculous disease before allowing the lung to re-expand. We actually continued for eighteen months; the lung re-expanded without difficulty, and her x-ray showed only residual scarring at the site of the cavity. Delores, who had become anxious about her own situation, accompanied her mother on her final visit. I repeated her x-ray; it was unchanged, again normal.

A year later real tragedy struck. I had been impressed with the relatively few cancers I had seen in our Indian patient population and had wondered, indeed, if these people had some resistance to the development of malignancies. But Emma developed a new series of symptoms. Studies at the hospital demonstrated an advanced cancer of the uterus, from which she died a few months later. Understandably, Delores was once again anxious, so, for reassurance more than anything, I repeated her chest x-ray. To my dismay I now saw a round nodule, about 2 centimeters in diameter, in her right lower lobe.

When unsuspected nodules are found in x-rays, particularly in older adults, whether smokers or not, the major conditions in the differential diagnosis are lung cancer or a solitary spread from another tumor, and benign conditions, including both inflammatory diseases and non-malignant tumors. The most important test one can do in this situation is attempt to unearth any prior x-rays and review them. I have already

128

stressed the mantra "Brains are good, but old films are better," and it surely applied here.

For Delores, I did not need to search. The two prior chest x-rays were right there in her x-ray folder. To my surprise, on the x-ray from one year before, the nodule was there, less than one centimeter in size, but in retrospect clearly visible. Despite my skill and the care with which I had studied the prior film, I had totally missed the abnormality! And her initial x-ray from three years previously? I saw what could have been a very tiny smudge at the same site. My own comparative study, along with the opinion of others to whom I showed the film, could only suggest that perhaps, just perhaps, it had been abnormal even back then.

But, more important, it was surely there now, apparently growing slowly. Despite her young age and apparent health, the question was raised, could it be a tumor? I have always taught that in biology and medicine the answer to "could it be" must always be "yes." A more appropriate question is, "what is the likelihood that a shadow represents a specific disorder?" It was essential for Delores that we know. Biopsy via a needle had not yet been done for shadows of this type. I arranged for thoracic surgery to be performed at the Indian Hospital at Shawnee, Oklahoma, where arrangements with surgeons from the Medical School in Oklahoma City had been made. The nodule was removed; under the microscope it proved to be a granuloma, the tissue reaction expected from tuberculosis. Delores recovered well and stayed well.

Mother and daughter had the same condition. In all likelihood Delores had caught the germ from her mother. A focus of primary pulmonary tuberculosis in her lower lobe, the common site for that stage of the disease, had failed to resolve and had grown.

Emma and her daughter illustrate many aspects of medicine in addition to the standard approach to a new tuberculous admission. The frequency of the disease in family members is perhaps most important.

Years later Gerald Baum and I reported a series of cases of similar enlarging nodules due to histoplasmosis. It appears that this variant of disease is more common in histo than it is in TB, and I wondered if Delores had had histoplasmosis rather than TB. I wrote to Bethesda Naval Hospital, where we had sent the pathologic material from her nodule, and raised the question. Their response was critical of me: they had stained the tissue for bacteria then, and it was full of tuberculosis germs, a fact I had forgotten!

Also years later, using a calculation known as doubling time, we were able to measure the growth rate of some tumors. We were amazed to learn that, when cancer of the lung occurs in solitary nodule form, it grows at a steady doubling time rate, rather than wildly and irregularly as one might expect. I used copies of Delores's x-rays for teaching and was able to demonstrate that the growth rate of her nodule was totally irregular, and thus, should not have represented a malignancy. Had we known that at the time, I am certain we still would have removed the nodule just to be safe. But our anxiety level—and hers—would surely have been much less!

Ella Marie

The situation for Ella Marie Farmer was quite different. She was older (sixty-five) and frailer; she had been ill for months, with cough and fatigue the prominent symptoms. Her chest x-ray revealed spotty disease throughout her entire left lung without an evident cavity. There may well have been one, simply obscured from my view. Her sputum was positive. An attempted pneumothorax was unsuccessful—an adequate free "space" could not be developed. I took advantage of her unilateral disease by employing another procedure: the phrenic "crush." The phrenic nerves, one on each side, run from the brain through the neck to supply the diaphragm, the large muscle separating the chest from the abdomen. When the phrenic nerve stimulates the diaphragm to contract, it descends, and a person takes a breath—air enters the lung. This phrenic nerve is easily accessible in the neck; a surgical procedure in which the nerve is literally crushed with a clamp results in temporary paralysis of the diaphragmatic leaflet on one side—the side of the diseased lung. When the diaphragm rises on that side, the lung is compressed; consequently, the work of breathing is done primarily by the healthy lung while the diseased one heals. The procedure can be supplemented by pneumoperitoneum, in which air is introduced into the peritoneal cavity with the result being that the flail diaphragmmatic leaflet rises even higher.

The evidence in favor of this procedure was not as good as for pneumothorax; in addition, it could affect the ability of the person to breathe, especially if their respiratory reserve was already limited. Hopefully, within six months the diaphragm had regained its normal function, although this did not always occur, and some residual weakness was common.

Nevertheless, for Ella Marie the procedure worked like a charm. Her sputum became negative, her strength returned, and she was able to be discharged from the sanatorium after being there just a bit more than a year.

Barney

Tuberculosis was quite prevalent among the Navajo Indians. The sick patients far outnumbered the beds available in Arizona and New Mexico necessary for their care. Many individuals, therefore, were transferred to facilities far away from their homes where specialized treatment was available. One such transferee under my care in Talihina was Barney Begay, a Navajo man in his late twenties. The specifics of his situation at the onset of his illness were unknown to me; by the time I managed him, his disease was stable. The right upper lobe of his lung was shrunken and scarred, with a large cavity occupying its central portion. The remainder of his lungs were clear of disease. Barney's sputum was consistently positive for tubercle bacilli. He coughed, especially at night, and his sputum was occasionally streaked with blood, but otherwise, his general condition was good. His records indicated he had received antituberculous medications in such a fashion that he was surely resistant to all of them. I did have the new drug, isoniazid, available, but I knew it to be rather unlikely that isoniazid alone could arrest his disease.

In this situation, thoracoplasty—surgery on the chest (thorax)— was indicated. Thoracoplasty was a standard operation for pulmonary

131

tuberculosis in the days before chemotherapy. It is the rib cage which keeps the lungs expanded to their full shape; if the ribs are not present, the pressure of gravity collapses the remaining chest wall inwards, and this, in turn, compresses and collapses the underlying lung. Thoracoplasty was the ideal procedure to force collapse and closure of upper lobe cavities, when other methods had failed, as in Barney's case.

Thoracoplasty was ordinarily performed in two or three separate operations to remove the upper five to seven ribs over the affected zone. The operations involved a moderate degree of blood loss. The price of thoracoplasty was permanent deformity of the chest, not entirely concealed by clothing, but the price was considered small by patients and physicians, if cure and release from years of hospitalization in a sanatorium could be achieved. The operation had a high rate of success if the patients were properly chosen, and if the function of their lungs was such that they could tolerate the loss of some breathing mechanics. In situations like Barney's, it offered an opportunity for cure.

The Eastern Oklahoma Tuberculosis Sanatorium, a state facility, was on a hill near the Indian Hospital. I was fortunate that the director there, Dr. F. P. Baker, was a skilled surgeon with a long and voluminous experience in thoracoplasty. While I was in Talihina, he was feted in Oklahoma City by a large group of his former patients, after he had successfully performed a total of *five thousand* stages of the operation!

Arrangements were easily made for him to operate on Barney at our hospital, and the two stages of the seven-rib procedure were without complication. I added isoniazid to his regimen before the first operation and continued it for some months afterwards. It was immensely gratifying to see Barney's sputum convert to negative for the TB germ for the first time in years. Later that year we were able to transfer him back to Arizona for discharge to his home.

Thoracoplasty was a major procedure, only applicable to a relatively small percentage of hospitalized patients. But for those whose situation called for it, and for whom the surgery was successful, thoracoplasty could be life-saving, albeit at the price of some deformity.

Change!

With the advent of isoniazid in the 1950s, the proper principles of modern chemotherapy were learned: prolonged uninterrupted treatment with multiple medicines to which the patient's organisms were susceptible. In addition, in the decade from the mid '50s until the early '60s, our long-standing basic principles of tuberculosis care were gradually modified after great hesitancy in some quarters. Prolonged strict bed rest was eliminated; sanatorium care was found to be no longer necessary, and the sanatoria gradually closed. But some physicians during this time were slower to adapt their practice to the new realities. The following story demonstrates that I was, indeed, one such physician.

The star of the 1958 baseball World Series was Red Schoendienst, the Milwaukee Braves' second baseman. Shortly thereafter, it was announced that Schoendienst had been diagnosed with tuberculosis. Al Silverman, a friend and sports writer, editing the 1959 issue of *Baseball Heroes*, called me in Michigan for my thoughts on Schoendienst's future. And there I am, in Howard Cohn's article *Can Schoendienst Come Back?*

> *In Schoendienst's case, his physicians are reluctant to discuss his baseball future until they know the extent of tissue damage and see how well he responds to treatment. But one distinguished outsider, Dr. Robert Green, a specialist in chest diseases at the Veterans Administration Hospital in Ann Arbor, Michigan, and an instructor at the University of Michigan medical school, believes it unlikely that Red will play again. "I can only speak from general experience, because I have not examined the patient," says Dr. Green, who is an avid baseball fan. "On this basis, though, Schoendienst has two things working against him. One is the danger of a relapse. The other is his age, which makes this danger more acute. If he were a younger man, I should think the chances would be good that after proper convalescence he'd be able to rejoin his team. But he is 36 now and will be 37 by the time anyone who has spoken so far holds out hope that he can be really active again. At his age, it will not be easy to work himself*

back into the strong physical condition demanded of a major-league athlete. He was in the twilight of his playing career before he even came down with the disease. For him to endanger his future health just to get one or two more playing years under his belt would seem to be very foolhardy.

My touch of national fame was tarnished by the fact that the magazine appeared on the stands in the spring of 1959, just as Schoendienst, fully active, opened the season playing with the Braves!

In this transitional era, advances in anesthesia and in surgical techniques, along with the medicines, permitted us also to consider an approach almost unthinkable, and rarely attempted, in prior times: actual surgical removal of diseased areas of lung. Initially our objective had been the closure and elimination of cavities. Now we could resect them or remove segments of lobes, entire lobes, or even entire lungs, as I have described above with Bette Sue.

That brings me to Joseph Brophy. A veteran of the Korean war, he had returned home, entered college, finished law school and had just joined a law firm when, one morning, while washing, he coughed and expectorated globs of blood. He promptly sought medical attention. An x-ray revealed a cavity in his right upper lobe, surrounded by multiple other spots, all of which was proven to be due to tuberculosis. I placed him at modified bed rest, then still a staple of therapy, and started an effective multidrug regimen. He—and I—were pleased with his rapid response; his cough cleared, his sputum became negative, and his x-ray showed rapid improvement. In those days it was common for us to evaluate the anatomic improvement by specialized x-rays called tomograms after about six months of treatment. With his rapid response, and at his urging because of his desire to return to work, I ordered the tomograms somewhat earlier. Unfortunately, the cavity was still present, though smaller and much thinner-walled. I discussed the options with Joe and, shortly thereafter, he underwent a surgical removal of two of the segments of his right upper lobe, those containing the cavity and the residual disease. Fortunately, the procedure was uneventful; he recovered rapidly, and after a few more months of chemotherapy, he was discharged to begin a productive career.

Although anyone would surely rate his result as positive, in one sense he was a victim of our attitudes of the time. By the end of the sixties decade, we knew that cavity closure was no longer essential; what mattered was the ability of our medications to eliminate the TB organism, that is, to turn the sputum negative and to keep it that way. In some patients thin-walled cavitary spaces persisted; no matter, if the course of treatment was completed, long-term control, without relapse, was ensured for the majority of patients.

Surgery?!

The decade of the 1960s was the heyday of resectional surgery for tuberculosis, as mentioned previously. It was a rare, almost forgotten, measure thereafter, not only by me, but generally. Then...

Byung Lee, originally from Korea, was a thirty-year-old graduate student at the University of Michigan. I saw her in our County TB clinic in 1995 with active tuberculosis. Her history was unusual. She had first been diagnosed with the disease, limited to her right upper lobe, as an undergraduate in Virginia. Treated with standard oral medicines, she had done well. It was unclear, however, if her original organism had been completely studied. This became important two years later when, while at Brown, her x-ray had worsened, and she was treated a second time, again with a satisfactory response. Now she had relapsed for the second time, again with shadows limited to her right upper lobe including a cavity. The TB germ we recovered was resistant to two of the major anti-TB medicines, and we postulated that she might have been initially resistant to at least one of them, a condition more common in Korea than here. I designed an effective re-treatment regimen, and once again she improved.

We did not find any evidence of a deficient immune system; the unusual double relapse was probably due to inadequate treatment. Yet I was greatly concerned. After six months of our medications her sputum was negative, but her x-ray had improved only slightly, with good evidence that the cavity was still present. She should remain well; but she

135

had been in the same situation twice previously and had relapsed. The rest of her lungs, carefully examined, were entirely normal. I thought it would be wise to remove the diseased right upper lobe, hopefully to prevent the unlikely, but possible, third relapse. She and our surgeons agreed but, as she was alone in this country, she asked if the surgery could be done at home in Seoul. From my work on an international committee, I happened to know a chest internist at a major hospital there, and I made arrangements with her.

Then what I feared might happen, did. My colleague notified me that the Korean surgeons were unimpressed with the residual x-ray findings. E-mails flew back and forth. I explained that my concern lay in the two prior relapses, more than in the x-ray appearance. Finally, my opinion prevailed, and the resection was carried out successfully. However, they failed to culture the operative specimen, so we remained uncertain of the resistance status of her organisms.

Byung returned to Ann Arbor. She was well; she completed her studies here and moved on to an academic career in the East. The last time I heard from her she was healthy and happy.

Byung's course was reminiscent to me of an earlier era, when multiple relapses predicted a grim prognosis. I was reminded of Byung when I recently read about a young man with TB and resistant organisms who, nevertheless, traveled to Europe on his honeymoon. His treatment, too, led to a surgical resection. Much concern has been rightfully expressed about the specter of the increasing prevalence of multiple drug resistant organisms in the world, as today chemotherapy is the mainstay of treatment. These two cases should encourage us to recall the lessons and procedures of the past when, despite the lack of effective medicines, we could, nonetheless, make headway against the white plague.

It is good not to forget those past lessons.

Variable Manifestations

The manifestations of tuberculosis are tremendously variable. The natural history of the infection depends on factors related to the germ itself, immune factors in the host, and their interrelationship. Sadly, despite many scientific advances, these factors remain for the most part poorly understood.

Tuberculosis is spread from one infected individual to others via the expectoration of the germs in what are termed "droplet nuclei." Not everyone who is exposed is infected; indeed, it ordinarily requires prolonged close contact to "catch" the disease. The illness resulting from this primary infection is usually entirely without symptoms, recognized only by a positive skin test. Whether or not the infection will then progress to disease, and the rate at which it may do so, is another variable. In a small percentage of individuals, especially those with compromised immune systems and those whose immune systems are still developing, namely children under the age of five, the primary infection can be severe, progressive and fatal. Although in everyone the organisms tend to spread throughout the body, they become quiescent and do not cause disease. The only apparent residual is a positive skin test; in this phase we call patients' status "latent tuberculosis." The illness, however, can recrudesce at any time. The lifetime risk for relapse is 10-15%, and half of this risk occurs in the first few years. To prevent such, it is policy today to treat latent tuberculosis with isoniazid. The majority of cases of tuberculosis seen in countries such as the United States, where the incidence of the disease is quite low, is due to breakdown of the theoretically healed residua of that long-distant primary infection; a second infection from a more recent contact can also occur. I present a few patients who illustrate these variations.

Time

Frank Walker was twenty-two, in the Army stationed in Germany, when he contracted a severe pneumonia in the lower lobe of his right lung. He was hospitalized and treated; he recovered and returned to duty. During his hospitalization multiple tests had been performed, including culture of his sputum, not only for the usual pneumonia-causing bacteria, but also for the TB germ. The reason for the TB culture was unclear, although since it was ordered on admission, it probably was because the diagnosis of Frank's exact illness may not have been certain then. In any case a single specimen grew out an organism which resembled the TB germ; the organism was injected into a guinea pig, which succumbed on schedule: it was the TB germ. (The chemical and genetic procedures we now have available which differentiate the TB germ from others in the same class were not then available.) These procedures took three months, at which time Walker was comfortably performing his regular military duties. He was recalled and transferred to the Army's specialized tuberculosis unit at Valley Forge in the United States.

There Walker appeared well, and his x-ray appeared normal. He was subjected to multiple tests looking for a possible site of infection. His tuberculin test (the skin test which demonstrates prior infection with the TB germ) was positive, but all his other tests were negative, including attempts to reculture the organism. After much discussion, it was decided the evidence was inadequate to establish a diagnosis of TB—perhaps, for example, specimens had been mixed up in the laboratory. Walker was discharged from the service.

Two years later a mini-film was taken at the factory at which Walker worked, but nothing was reported about it. But two years after that Walker suddenly expectorated blood. He was hospitalized at our Veterans hospital. His x-ray showed a large tuberculous cavity in his right upper lobe, his sputum revealed the TB germ, and the diagnosis of active tuberculosis was established.

We obtained and reviewed all of Walker's prior records and x-rays. In a bronchogram, one of the specialized tests he had undergone at Valley Forge, in which dye is put into the lungs to examine the bronchi, my review showed a tiny nodule, less than one centimeter in size, in the right upper lobe. And the factory film showed a much larger nodule at the same site; the cavity was a further progression of that lesion.

Could that tiny nodule four years earlier have been responsible for the positive TB culture? By itself, it would have been rare for a spot of that size to do so; but perhaps, we postulated, the pneumonia had caused a significant production of sputum; a few germs from the nodule had been swept up into the pneumonic sputum and produced the positive culture.

Walker responded well to treatment, and his disease was controlled. But the point worth highlighting is that, in contrast to many other cases, it took four full years for Walker's disease to progress from a very tiny lesion to a cavity and symptomatic illness.

The time frame in Antoinette Cebelak's story is even longer. She was a little girl in the early years of the 20th century in what is now Slovakia, when her grandmother, who lived with her and her parents, developed a fatal case of tuberculosis. Antoinette apparently became infected, because she was sent to a preventorium, a facility in which it was hoped children would not have their potential illness progress to disease. It was evidently successful; she returned home to live normally.

Antoinette later immigrated to the United States, married and had children. In the latter years of the 20th century, in her ninth decade of life, she visited a grandson here in Ann Arbor. She was noted to be coughing; evaluation revealed the presence of active tuberculosis; treatment was begun promptly. We evaluated the family and discovered that her two-year-old great-granddaughter had a positive tuberculin skin test. Fortunately, the child had no disease, but we treated her latent infection. That treatment should prevent progression to disease, presumably forever. Then again, who can say for certain? When that child is elderly, and her general immunity wanes, the dormant organism may once again develop a new lease on life. A disease we can trace to the 19th century, and Antoinette's grandmother, might cast its influence well into the 21st century, fully six generations later.

Florence Gann's story is in marked contrast. She was seventeen when she was brought to the hospital in extremis. Her mother claimed she had been entirely well six weeks previously, when the family had visited an uncle known to have TB, who had left another hospital against advice. She had been febrile for two weeks and then had failed rapidly. Her x-ray showed extensive bilateral tuberculosis in a form simulating pneumonia. Her sputum was heavily positive, but before I could institute effective treatment, she had died. It is theoretically possible she had been infected previously, but this history and course suggested recent primary infection. With good reason the form of her disease was termed "galloping consumption." Like the young boy I had seen in medical school with tuberculous meningitis, and in strong contrast to Walker and Cebelak, this extreme rapidity of course exemplifies the temporal variability of the disease.

Ramirez—A Routine and a Lesson

Theodore Ramirez was a full-blooded San Ildefonso Indian. The San Ildefonso are a New Mexico Pueblo tribe; I never learned why Ted lived in northern Oklahoma. No matter—he had been ill for some months with malaise, cough and sputum production, including hemoptysis, when admitted in May 1952. His x-ray showed extensive infiltrates all through the left lung, which was contracted in size, with a slight shift of the heart towards that side. He was febrile, looked quite ill, and weighed only 100 pounds. His sputum was heavily positive for tubercle bacilli. I did not yet have a supply of isoniazid, the recently discovered wonder drug, but I probably would not have used it anyway, since I was just learning about it. I put Ramirez at complete bed rest and started him on the standard regimen of streptomycin, one gram daily by injection, and 12 grams of PAS orally each day. I fully expected this treatment to be successful.

By mid July after six weeks of treatment, Theodore had not improved. He was still spiking temperatures, and had continued to lose weight, now down to 94 pounds. I thought that in all likelihood his TB germ must have been initially resistant to streptomycin; adding isoniazid was clearly the intervention to make. Before I did so, recalling Charlie Vandenbosch from my residency, I ordered another chest x-ray as a baseline, a routine which I now worshipped. I knew that it was better to control each change in management with a timely film.

Surprise! Ramirez's x-ray showed a large spontaneous pneumothorax on the left; his lung was adherent to the chest wall at the apex, but was otherwise 80% collapsed. The heart had now shifted to the right, and a few patchy infiltrates involved the right lung. The lower half of the pleural space was filled with fluid, an air-fluid level at its surface.

I inserted a needle into the chest; the air pressure was positive; the fluid, of which I removed a pint, was thick pus full of tubercle bacilli. Ted had a bronchopleural fistula, a direct connection from the diseased lung to the pleural space. I added isoniazid to his regimen, and shortly thereafter, reduced his streptomycin to twice weekly.

I questioned Ramirez vigorously regarding a change in symptoms, particularly chest pain. His English was better than many of my patients; he denied any change, and a review of the nurses notes over the previous six weeks also showed no mention of a change in his symptoms.

Ramirez promptly felt better, and his improvement persisted. I tapped his chest weekly, often removing fluid and air each time. By December, after five months, his intrathoracic pressure became negative, which is normal. His lungs cleared considerably, and his heart and mediastinum regained their shift to the left. His sputum cultures became negative. The air fluid level, which represented pus in the chest, persisted for six months; the air was gone after another three, leaving him with a small lung and, surprisingly, only mildly thickened pleura. INH was discontinued after a year; SM and PAS continued for another year. With only some residual shortness of breath with exertion, at a weight of 133, Ramirez was discharged as "arrested" after two years of hospitalization. At follow up two years later he was stable.

I had been taught that in the pre-chemotherapy era a tuberculous bronchopleural fistula such as Ramirez had was often fatal. It absolutely required immediate surgical drainage with a large bore chest tube, and the infection was usually mixed, with ordinary bacteria in addition to the TB bacillus. The fact that Ramirez's lung was adherent at the apex, thus preventing complete collapse of his lung, was surely helpful to him. However, the main lesson I learned was that chemotherapy, particularly isoniazid, was an immensely powerful tool; when accompanied by judicious use of frequent thoracenteses (removal of the pleural fluid and air), surgery might neither be necessary nor desirable.

Ramirez wrote an unsolicited laudatory letter about me to the Bureau of Indian Affairs, a copy of which was forwarded to me. I was quite pleased with the kind words.

Emergency!

Claude Rivers, ¾ Cherokee, fifty-one years old, was a big, big man, weighing well over 200 pounds. He had been coughing for over a year, but for the last three weeks or so, he had had chest pain and severe shortness of breath. He was also hoarse, and had right lower quadrant pain. When he arrived his lips and fingernails were blue, indicating oxygen lack. His x-ray showed a left hydropneumothorax (air and fluid in the left pleural space) with 60% collapse of a left lung in which I could see two large cavities and, fortunately, only a few patches of disease on the right. I tapped him immediately, removing 700 cc of air to attempt to equalize the pleural pressures and relieve his shortness of breath and shortly thereafter, I drew off 1375 cc of pus. These were literally acute lifesaving actions.

Tuberculous bronchopleural fistula with empyema (pus in the chest), which this was, was not only an emergency, but also likely to be fatal; but I had learned from Theodore Ramirez that death was not always the outcome. While chemotherapy with dihydrostreptomycin, isoniazid and PAS began its work on his extensive pulmonary, pleural, laryngeal and, probably, intestinal tuberculosis, I began mine with the needle. Two days later I withdrew 200 cc of pus; the next day he was worse, and at his bed rather than the treatment room, I removed a liter of air. Claude began to improve. His major complaint soon shifted to his hemorrhoids!

Meanwhile, over the next two months, even as the fistula began to close and the residual air began to absorb, the fluid level rose. It required multiple taps to remove large amounts—an estimated total of four liters—of purulent TB-positive fluid. The predominant white blood cells in the fluid suggested a mixed infection; the streptomycin may have taken care of any non-TB bacilli there. My last successful tap in this initial period was after two months of treatment, after which his x-ray showed a persistent lateral air space, with marked thickening of the two layers of pleura—the visceral, covering the lung surface, and the parietal, on the inside of the chest wall.

In my chapter on pneumothorax in Gerald Baum's *Textbook On Pulmonary Diseases*, I wrote that the cause of an illness depends, in part, on where you are. I was thinking of Theodore, Claude and others. In the general population, spontaneous pneumothorax usually has no specific cause, whereas in the Indian Bureau, tuberculosis was its cause more often than not. This principle is now termed "context specificity."

Claude was the kind of patient for whom, as a doctor, one obviously did much more than just prescribe medicines. A secondary incident related to his case occurred a year or so later. Rashes were a bane of the doctor's life in the sanatorium. I saw multiple varieties, one more mysterious than the next. They came and went, ointments or no. Claude developed a peculiar spot on his right thigh, which ulcerated and wouldn't go away. I thought it might, in fact, be a basal cell carcinoma (a form of skin cancer) in an unusual location, so one day I removed it and sent it off to the lab in Bethesda. The report came back: blastomycosis!!—an uncommon fungus infection. I rechecked, but all the rest of Claude's disease was definitively tuberculosis, and nothing else. Still the cutaneous Blasto was a big surprise.

After a year of hospitalization and treatment Claude's sputum was still positive for tubercle bacilli. His fluid recurred, this time much clearer on tap and not purulent. (It probably was an "ex vacuo" effusion: the thick pleura prevented the lung from completely expanding; the pressures in the pleural space became highly negative, and eventually fluid exuded.) I transferred him to the Shawnee sanatorium, closer to Oklahoma City, where arrangements had been made for University surgeons to operate on our patients. A year and a half after his initial admission, Claude underwent a complete left pneumonectomy for residual cavitary disease in a pretty well destroyed left lung. Except for post operative hepatitis, he did well, and was eventually discharged.

Claude was yet another case in which tuberculous bronchopleural fistula proved not to be fatal. But it certainly made for some excitement and a major feeling of accomplishment during those first few days of urgent treatment.

Patsy and BCG

BCG is a vaccine against tuberculosis. The letters stand for Bacillus (of) Calmette Guerin, the names of the two French investigators who developed the vaccine. In the 1920's they took a bovine strain of the TB bacillus and passed it through many laboratory culturing procedures. The germ evolved into one that, while still alive, did not possess the ability to kill the animals into which it was injected; instead, it increased their ability to withstand subsequent infection with the tuberculosis germ itself when challenged.

BCG underwent hundreds of trials in humans. Although the results were variable, most international authorities accepted that it had some value. BCG did not, and does not, prevent subsequent infection with the TB germ, but in countries or municipalities where there was a high incidence of tuberculosis, the use of the vaccine in uninfected individuals could help prevent the serious and often fatal complications should infection occur. Such dreaded events could develop, especially in children recently infected by the germ.

Some of the most important studies on BCG had been performed in the United States by Joseph Aronson and his colleagues from the Henry Phipps Institute in Philadelphia. The experiments had involved American Indians and Alaskan natives and had shown favorable results. Dr. Robert Saylor, who was my mentor at the sanatorium in Albuquerque, New Mexico had worked with Aronson. My knowledge about BCG was thus stimulated.

Besides the doubt in some quarters as to its effectiveness, BCG had a downside. The organism had the ability to provoke the reaction to skin tests used for the diagnosis of tuberculosis. In localities of high TB prevalence this made little difference, as most of the population was infected anyway. The positive skin test and possible diagnostic confusion was a minor price to pay for the protection it offered to the multitudes, who might otherwise become infected with the TB germ, but not succumb. On the other hand, where TB was less common and the skin test more important in diagnosis, BCG could diminish its diagnostic value. This was one reason the vaccine achieved little popularity in the United States; more important, later studies by Comstock from Johns Hopkins reported that the vaccine was not helpful here.

Today, with much immigration to the U.S. from parts of the world where BCG vaccination remains common, physicians regularly deal with this diagnostic confusion. The positive skin test due to BCG wanes with time, as—perhaps—does the relative immunity it confers; a positive test in an adult who received BCG as a child almost invariably indicates subsequent infection with the TB germ. Many individuals, however, have been told and/or believe that their positive skin test is due to the BCG, rather than the supervening TB infection. They are hard to convince that they risk subsequent development of disease.

After I delivered my first baby in Talihina I was surprised to see the nurse give the newborn an injection. When I asked about it, I was told it was the Indian Bureau policy to "inject all newborns with BCG." (This was prior to Comstock's report.) While this surprised me, I understood the reasons why; however, I was later disturbed to learn that the policy did not include follow-up with any of these children to see if, indeed, their skin tests had become positive, or if a rare complication had ensued.

One such infant who was born in our hospital, and who, therefore, received the BCG at birth, was a half-blood Choctaw girl, Patsy. She was illegitimate, and the whereabouts of her mother later unknown. Her grandmother was dead, so she was cared for by her great-grandmother, who was not an elderly woman. At ten months of age, Patsy was brought to the hospital after three days of vomiting and severe diarrhea. She was admitted, febrile, lethargic and dehydrated. Her weight fell to nineteen pounds. She did not improve with her initial standard management of hydration and anti-diarrheals.

Our technician suggested that he had seen amoebae in her stool; a diagnosis of amebic colitis was not unreasonable. The recommended treatment at that time was an arsenic-containing compound; unfortunately, tiny Patsy was prescribed adult doses of this potentially toxic medication by a young, poorly trained colleague. At first, she may have improved a bit, but then her fever recurred, and her condition worsened with evidence of kidney and liver damage. Her weight fell further to 13 pounds 8 ounces, despite swollen hands and feet. At this point, almost two months after admission, a chest x-ray was taken. It showed innumerable little spots scattered throughout the lungs, a condition characteristic of a state known as miliary tuberculosis. This is one of the most feared forms of TB, in which the germs, spreading throughout the blood stream, pepper the lungs with thousands of organisms. Not surprisingly, it was uniformly fatal in the days before chemotherapy.

I transferred Patsy to the TB floor. She was a very, very sick little girl. I started treatment with the two powerful anti-TB drugs available, stretomycin and isoniazid, both by injection. The feared further complication of TB meningitis did not occur; gradually, so very gradually, Patsy began to improve. It took almost eight months before she became a more normal little girl.

We did our regular contact evaluation to ascertain the source of Patsy's infection. Patsy's great-grandma was negative, as was one other fairly regular visitor to their home. The source of her infection remained unknown.

Or did it? Unfortunately, in one sense, all my attempts to culture the TB germ from Patsy failed. Such is not unusual for the miliary form of tuberculosis, as organisms are not eliminated from the body in large numbers like they are in the ordinary cases of pulmonary tuberculosis. Perhaps some unknown casual contact with an active case had occurred. But in my mind, another possibility existed: the BCG. Remember, BCG is a live, albeit attenuated, organism. The arsenic toxicity, plus her diarrheal illness, had severely depressed all her functions and bodily defenses, including that of the immune system. It is not far-fetched to posit that, under these harrowing circumstances, the BCG organism had grown, overcoming whatever defenses remained, and spread through her tiny body. Other documented instances of this sort of tragedy are on record from all over the world. I never had any proof, but I felt Patsy's situation was an example of a rare, but dire, complication of the BCG vaccination in an immunocompromised host.

Eventually I discontinued the practice of BCG injections for newborns at our hospital.

I revisited Talihina with my family eight years later to visit old friends we had made there. I asked, with some trepidation, about Patsy. One of them knew her. "She's alive and well," he reported, but "you know, she's not a pretty little girl"—as if I cared about that! Clearly her strengths lay elsewhere: that once pitiable infant had not only recovered, but was a true survivor!

Pieta

I made the diagnosis right there in the clinic room. They presented quite a tableau: Virginia sat in the center of the room, head bowed over her baby, holding it in her arms; but the baby, Hinnie Jean, was stretched out, rigid, stiff. I approached; I could not turn the baby's neck, in which I also felt enlarged lymph nodes. She was feverish, thin, wasted. Virginia said she had been this way, nursing poorly, lethargic, for the last two of the sixteen months of her life. My diagnostic test was simple: I took Virginia—not Hinnie Jean—to the x-ray room, and there it was: a large tuberculous cavity in the left upper lung with spread elsewhere. Hinnie Jean had caught tuberculosis from her mother; she now had tuberculous meningitis, TB of the lining of the brain and spinal cord.

Virginia, a pretty twenty-five-year-old Seminole woman, had herself been coughing for a couple of months, her sputum occasionally streaked with blood, but she felt relatively well and was only concerned with her baby. I hospitalized them both.

Hinnie Jean weighed only seventeen pounds. Her right eyelid drooped, the right side of her body was more rigid than the left with spontaneous seizures of her right arm. Her chest x-ray showed swollen lymph glands at the root of her right lung; I smeared the secretions from her throat and demonstrated the TB germ. More to the point, I tapped her spinal fluid. Usually crystal clear, this fluid was cloudy, full of inflammatory cells, low sugar and elevated protein—the typical findings of TB. I cultured the TB germ from it. I promptly instituted treatment with isoniazid and streptomycin—the best available drugs—by injection into her muscles, and the streptomycin repeatedly into the spinal fluid itself. We fed her by tube and by subcutaneous injection of fluids. It was rough going, and it took more than two months before I could claim she was improving. Her spinal fluid cleared very gradually; after a year it still contained a few inflammatory cells, with elevated protein and low sugar. She began to walk, with a spastic paralysis of her right side. I have a picture of her, a chubby little girl, sitting with Amos and Patsy, two other hospitalized children.

Meanwhile Virginia responded well to treatment. After a year her left upper lung was removed surgically. She was discharged from the hospital two years after her admission with her now three-year-old. I have no follow-up information about Hinnie Jean; but she had certainly come a long way from that first tableau I have in my mind of her as a tiny infant, stretched out rigidly in her mother's arms.

VA Records

A great source of diagnostic information is the prior medical record. Today, surprisingly, the record itself is often neglected, because of a tendency for the narrative summary of a hospitalization or doctor-patient contact to replace the record itself. But some findings, seemingly minor, can be omitted in the summary. Perhaps even more often, transcription errors hide results that may figure prominently in later problems. Years ago, in the Veterans Administration, summaries were often short—true summaries rather than narrative descriptions—so that the record itself required more careful review. At times, however, prior records, for example of hospitalizations at other sites, were inadequately collected and included.

Two other collections of data were helpful for those who were aware of them. One was called the Claims folder, kept in a Regional Office of the Veterans Administration. A file existed for any veteran who had ever submitted any sort of claim. It included not only a copy of the claim, but also information related to it, including service records and reports of hospitalizations. A third file was the Correspondence folder. Also kept at a regional office, it included, as its name implies, all correspondence from and to the veteran, and often included letters from other related parties. This information could sometimes shed light on a particular problem.

More sinned against...

I found a letter in the original Polish, as well as the English translation, in one man's correspondence folder. I reproduce it here as best as I can remember after all these years, knowing that I fail to capture the primal pathos.

Dear President Truman,

How could you do such a thing? Here is my son, a cripple because of the war and what you did to him, he can't work, he can't do anything any more, he just sits at home. She works but what can she earn so they are starving. He is a hero and you should be giving him more money than you do so what do you do instead but take money away from him. It is a terrible terrible thing. For this he went to the army and the jungle for the war? Shame shame. I am mad and I cry.

It was signed Mrs. Stanislaw Szczepanski.

The response to her letter was as follows:

Dear Mrs. Szczepanski,

I have read your letter and I am ashamed too. I have asked my assistant, Mr. Clark Clifford, to check into your son's case. If what you say is confirmed I will see that the injustice is corrected and that the people responsible are reprimanded.

Thank you for writing to me,

> *Sincerely yours,*
> *Harry S Truman*
> *President of the United States*

With that introduction, let me jump ahead eleven years, from 1949 to 1960, when Arthur Suppan, the son in question, was admitted to my tuberculosis ward at the VA Hospital in Ann Arbor. (He had anglicized his name.) Known to have had tuberculosis deemed connected to his military service in World War II, now a major pulmonary hemorrhage portended relapse. I found an emaciated man, the left side of his body scarred and markedly disfigured. His chest x-ray revealed why: he had a large cavity in his right upper lobe with multiple patchy spots all through the right lung. But, on the left side virtually no lung was visible. A thoracoplasty—the most extensive I had ever seen—had been performed. This operation was typically done in stages, removing usually two, sometimes three, ribs at a time for a total removal of five, six, or seven ribs—rarely more. In Suppan's case, major portions of *eleven* of the twelve ribs had been partially removed, leaving him, quite literally, a shell of a man.

There was another unusual aspect to his chest x-ray. At the very base of his left lung I saw a thick dense shadow along the side and at the back of his chest. It had the typical characteristics of a pleural plaque, a thickening of dense scar tissue which obliterated the space between the outer lining of the lung and the inner lining of the chest cage. Could it have been the result of bleeding into the pleural space at the time of his surgery? I had wondered why eleven ribs had been removed. Could the shadow have been there before the operation and misdiagnosed as part of his lung TB?

The unraveling of Suppan's case was clearly going to take time, as it apparently dated back to his wartime service, and the history he gave us included prior hospitalizations and treatment. Right now his sputum was heavily positive for the TB germ; we learned later, fortunately, that his organism was still susceptible to our major anti-TB drugs, and treatment was begun. Meanwhile, my detective work also began. I reviewed his extensive service medical records and his claim and correspondence records, where I found the President Truman correspondence, as well as records from other hospitals and administrations. I was thrilled as each piece of the puzzle began to fall into place.

Arthur Suppan was twenty-three years old in the winter of 1939, when he had a severe case of presumed influenza. He told us he spent the entire winter in bed, only eventually improving in the spring. He received no medical care during this period. In 1941, before the war began, he was drafted into the Army. I obtained his induction chest x-ray—a mini film the size of a playing card—and it showed the pleural plaque, larger and thicker than seventeen years later. The film was presumably interpreted as normal, as Suppan was accepted into service: error # 1. (These little films were often on rolls of 500 or more; reading them was a horrendous task; errors, found retrospectively, were not uncommon.)

Then, in the South Pacific in the summer of 1943, Suppan developed fever, chest pain, and cough now with expectoration of blood. He improved somewhat with treatment, but TB was suspected, especially as his skin test was positive. Multiple studies, however, failed to demonstrate the TB germ; a positive skin test can often indicate infection with the TB germ, but without disease. His x-ray showed a shadow at the base of the left lung thought to be pneumonia: error # 2. It did not change, however, over seven months of hospitalization and observation, which included multiple studies, such as bronchoscopy (a lighted tube is passed and the bronchi, the lung airways, examined) and bronchography, in which dye is placed into the bronchial tree to exam it. Suppan was finally diagnosed with chronic bronchitis, and chronic pneumonia: error # 3. He was discharged from the service in January, 1944. He returned to the states, married and started a family. An x-ray in 1945 was unchanged, but in the spring of 1946, Suppan's fever, weight loss and cough with blood spitting recurred. Suppan was then hospitalized at a major municipal tuberculosis hospital, where his x-ray now showed a tuberculous cavity at the top of the left lung and a dense shadow at the left base. His tuberculosis having developed within three years of discharge, in addition to his illness while in the Army, were administratively sufficient enough to connect the illness to his service, and financial compensation was begun.

Meanwhile, Suppan's sputum was positive for the TB germ and remained so; an attempt at artificial pneumothorax, a temporary procedure to attempt to collapse the cavity (which requires an intact pleural space) was unsuccessful. After a year of failure to respond, in 1947, just at the dawn of the streptomycin era, thoracoplasty was recommended. Error

4—the worst of them all—unfortunately lay in the interpretation that this shadow at the base indicated the need to remove all or portions of *eleven* ribs, instead of the usual maximum seven ribs. The procedure was probably successful, but Suppan, perhaps horrified by the physical result, left the sanatorium against advice before adequate evaluation and postoperative treatment could be accomplished.

Over the next two years occasional x-rays were strongly suggestive of relapse, with disease now in the right lung. Suppan, now unable to work and living in relative poverty, adamantly refused to cooperate with the public health authorities. In 1949 his fourteen-month-old son was hospitalized and died with tuberculous meningitis, undoubtedly transmitted from his father. The payments a veteran receives depend not only on his degree of disability, but also on the number of his dependents. Suppan now had only two dependents, his wife and remaining child, so his compensation was reduced. And it was this action that occasioned his mother's letter to the President.

I assume Clark Clifford determined the facts; I found no information in the records about any follow-up action or correspondence. I would guess that everyone's sympathy may well have been altered when the facts became known that the child had died due to having been infected by his father.

The rest of the story is more mundane. By the time Suppan was under my care in 1960, effective chemotherapy with anti-tuberculosis drugs was available. Despite complications of an allergic reaction to streptomycin, gastrointestinal intolerance to PAS, and recurrent nonspecific respiratory infections, we were able to stabilize Suppan and convert his sputum to negative. He gained weight, if only a few pounds. He was discharged, his disease quiescent, after twenty-one months of hospitalization. Unfortunately, he was promptly lost to follow-up, and whether his disease remained under control, or whether his pleural plaque was ever again misinterpreted, I do not know.

The most tragic aspect of Suppan's case is that he received multiple misdiagnoses of his pleural plaque. I remain surprised and upset by it, as the shadow is one of the few in radiology that is absolutely characteristic and should be unmistakable.

Deja vu

During the decade of the 1950s we learned just how powerful the drug isoniazid was. It could be used not only for treatment of active cases, but also for preventing the progression of tuberculous infection to tuberculous disease. We developed a list of high risk situations in which prophylactic therapy, today termed treatment of latent tuberculosis, was highly recommended. Prime examples were situations in which the body's immunity was compromised by illness or by certain medications. Unfortunately, but not surprisingly, the general medical community was slow to adopt this approach.

The rheumatologists referred Oscar Stuckey in 1962. A twenty-eight-year-old black man, they had diagnosed him with lupus erythematosus. This disease, then thought to be uncommon in blacks and men, involves the joints and connective tissues. They were about to begin treatment with steroids; however, they noted Oscar also had a positive tuberculin skin test; his chest x-ray was normal. They requested our opinion.

Even as early as 1962 this was a "no brainer" for me. Steroid therapy was classically known to depress the immune status. I strongly recommended Stuckey be given isoniazid while undergoing steroid treatment. This would prevent the tuberculous infection from progressing to active disease while his immune system was compromised. The rheumatologists were more concerned about the increased incidence of allergic reactions in lupus patients, and they declined to follow my recommendation. Six months later Oscar had widespread bilateral tuberculosis in his lungs, requiring prolonged hospitalization and treatment to control. His case was, regrettably, not the only one, nor the only disorder, in which we saw this distressing outcome, but the rapidity with which the disease spread was so striking that I used his case in my teachings to emphasize this point for many years.

Thirty years later in 1992, Jeanne Perkins was referred to our clinic. She had had painful and progressive rheumatoid arthritis for many years. A new class of disease-modifying agents (blockers of the protein tumor necrosis factor, which, among other actions, promoted inflammation) had been created. These agents also had serious immune-depressing

153

side effects. Jeanne had a family history of TB, a known positive skin test, and abnormal scars in her chest x-ray; despite these factors her rheumatologist prescribed one of the new agents, but without isoniazid coverage. Jeanne paid the price: in less than a month she became ill with miliary tuberculosis, a once fatal form of the disease, which spreads through the blood stream. Once again, it took prolonged treatment to bring her disease under control. It was Deja vu all over again. The need for isoniazid in TB-positive patients who are undergoing other immune-depressing treatments is clear. Sadly, this principle still requires emphasis.

Extrapulmonary TB

Tuberculosis can affect any organ in the body. I have already presented patients in whom the disease involved the lymph nodes, the pleural space, the meninges and the peritoneal cavity. A common and painful form involves the spine.

Ordinarily—but

Melvin Couchman, a thirty-three-year-old laborer, came to the hospital for back pain. His distress wasn't in the usual low back area, but higher up. An x-ray showed destructive lesions of the 10th and 11th thoracic vertebrae. They had collapsed onto each other, with the interspace between them destroyed, such that a casual perusal might suggest one large vertebra, rather than two reduced in size. Adjacent to these bones was a dense oblong structure on both sides, indicative of a paravertebral abscess. The x-ray was strongly suggestive of Pott's disease—tuberculosis of the spine. His skin test for TB was positive. Nothing pointed to an alternate diagnosis; chemotherapeutic treatment for tuberculosis was begun.

The tuberculosis germ enters through the respiratory tract; from there, in almost all individuals, it spreads through the body without causing disease as these distant foci heal. They may, however, break down later anywhere in the body. In Melvin's case this relapse had occurred in the spine.

A month or so into treatment, Melvin began to experience progressive left-sided chest pain. Physical examination and an x-ray revealed shadows, indicating fluid in the left pleural space, surrounding the lung—a pleural effusion. This was distinctly unusual. Sometimes, early in the course of tuberculosis, a pleural effusion may develop and heal, and later, an increased incidence of TB of the spine may be noted. But the reverse, a pleural effusion following established spinal disease, was almost unheard of. I reasoned that the abscess surrounding his vertebra might have ruptured into his chest. I aspirated the fluid. Unlike the clear fluid seen early in the disease, this fluid was scant, dark and cloudy, supporting my hypothesis.

Now in those days, standard practice for management of a paravertebral abscess was to leave it alone, expecting that with medical treatment and sometimes surgical spinal fusion for the bone disease, it would also heal. But this unusual situation suggested to me that drainage of the abscess would be a desirable approach to prevent further contamination of the chest cavity.

The young staff surgeon in orthopedics had recently completed his training. I presented my recommendation to him. He indicated they did not ordinarily believe in draining these abscesses, no matter the special circumstances. I asked that he discuss the case with his attending physician; the response was similar. Frustrated, I learned that the Chief of Orthopedics, Dr. Carl Badgely, a man with great experience in spinal tuberculosis, held Saturday morning clinics. I went and presented Melvin to him. Dr. Badgely repeated that, ordinarily, they did not drain paravertebral abscesses, but that it seemed to him a reasonable approach in this case. His younger colleagues now nodded in agreement. Triumphant, I was about to leave when Dr. Badgely asked me which medicine I thought had led to the greatest advance in the treatment of Pott's disease. As I mentioned each of the few anti-TB medicines available at that time, I was surprised to find him shaking his head. The answer, he said, was penicillin—which had no activity against the TB germ. But, in prior years, when they attempted surgery on Pott's disease patients, particularly children, they were foiled by the post-operative complication of staphylococcal skin infections, which penetrated deeply, and were serious if not fatal. Penicillin had permitted spinal surgery to proceed successfully!

When Melvin was then operated upon, I learned another reason why the surgery was rarely recommended. Instead of a large tense abscess, a dense area of extreme inflammation with only a small amount of actual pus was found. The inflammatory area densely adhered to the surrounding tissues, including the aorta. The surgeon did what he could, completing the operation. Fortunately, Melvin's recovery then proceeded as we had originally hoped, with stabilization of his spine and healing.

His situation taught me much and gave me the opportunity to consult with one of Michigan's historically great surgeons. His "ordinarily, but" reminded me of Dr. Colp's decision during my internship not to perform a colostomy on a woman in light of the patient's and her brother's history. Sometimes it takes a great and confident man to be willing to deviate from the standard approach.

Another one of the Greats

Vincent Scruggs was another patient I cared for with Pott's disease. A complication in his case led to my encounter with another Michigan great.

The first manifestation of Vincent's spinal tuberculosis was striking and remarkable. While still in his twenties he noted progressive back pain and fevers about which he did nothing. He then developed pain in his left groin, which became severe and led his thigh to flex up towards his abdomen. Eventually, his skin burst just below the groin with drainage of purulent material. X-rays demonstrated destruction of multiple thoracic vertebrae in his lower chest with the adjacent dense shadows of a paravertebral abscess. A catheter was gingerly introduced into the open wound in his groin; it easily advanced *eight inches* into his body. Dye was then injected, and x-rays were taken. Upon examination of the x-rays, the dye was seen to have traveled all the way up the iliopsoas muscle to the paravartebral abscess on both sides of his lower thoracic spine! The x-ray was surely one of the most remarkable in my experience.

Scruggs had then had multiple hospitalizations and courses of chemotherapy elsewhere with intermittent healing, then a reopening of his sinus tract, and an unsuccessful spinal fusion operation. When he was hospitalized on my service, he was a short, hunched over, unhappy man; his complaints were persistent back pain, fatigue and depression.

We were able to culture the drainage for the TB germ; laboratory tests showed it was resistant to all the major drugs available at the time except for two: viomycin (VM) and pyrazinamide (PZA). Initially I withheld these until I, after consultation with the orthopedic surgeons and others, could develop a long-term plan for his care. A few weeks later, however, Vincent told me of new symptoms: he had abruptly lost sensation and movement in his legs. I knew this development represented a surgical emergency. Scruggs was experiencing so-called Pott's paraplegia—paralysis of the lower half of his body due to the pressure of the abscesses around the vertebrae on his spinal cord. Rapid surgical drainage and relief of the pressure were essential.

It took a full morning on the telephone to get the orthopedic surgeons and the neurosurgeons to agree to operate jointly and to schedule the operation for later that day. I started the VM and PZA and waited in the surgical suite for the surgeons to appear. To my surprise, it was Eddie Kahn, the famous and legendary Chief of Neurosurgery at the University, one of the pioneers in the field, who appeared with his resident. The orthopedists were nowhere in sight. For the first time in many years, I scrubbed to help on the case, contributing little but retractor holding to the procedure. It was a long evening for all of us. Kahn found few remaining anatomical landmarks; he commented continuously during his dissection, at times profanely; he feared he was cutting across sinus tracts in the remarkably distorted tissues. He did the best he could, but he completed the surgery uncertain that he had relieved the pressure. Fortunately, he apparently had; post-operatively, Vincent's paralysis resolved. The added medications, with the help of the surgery, appeared

157

to be effective, because the drainage ceased. And some months later, true to form, Vincent once again left the hospital.

Scruggs's situation was a sad one; but it at least afforded me the pleasure and privilege of having worked with Dr. Kahn, who was able to offer Scruggs some relief, although who knows for how long.

Today

TB clinic

Most of my life has been spent taking care of people with tuberculosis. I saw my first cases in medical school and lived through the era of progress, when chemotherapy changed the disease from a tragedy to a curative illness. I continued that career after I retired from other activities, as I headed the local tuberculosis clinic in Washtenaw County, Michigan. If you think our practice today is nothing like the old days, you would be correct. Most of our clients are people with positive skin tests without disease, so-called latent tuberculosis; we now have guidelines to help decide whom to treat, so that much of the clinic work seems cut and dried. Once in a while, however, a single evening clinic is challenging, and I report on one.

Previously, my most unusual clinic had been geographic rather than clinical: the patients had originated from fourteen different countries! The problems this particular night were medical; besides a few "routine" cases of latent tuberculosis, I saw a new case of Pott's disease—tuberculosis of the spine—in an elderly black American man—and the two-month follow-up case of another patient with Pott's disease, also in an elderly black American man. Two cases of Pott's disease in one clinic must be very rare today anywhere in the United States. I saw a young Somali woman whose skin test conversion had been ignored in another state. She then developed "galloping consumption," rapidly spreading pulmonary tuberculosis, which had responded beautifully to treatment;

at this clinic, after nine months, she had completed therapy, and I (reluctantly) discontinued it. I saw a young Chinese woman treated originally in West Virginia without sputum having been collected. Now she had relapsed, and her germ was resistant to both isoniazid and streptomycin, and had probably been so originally. Treatment was complicated by severe liver toxicity. Now, after nine months, she was doing well. As her treatment program had been with less effective "second line" medications, I told her we needed to continue for a total of eighteen months. She and her husband were unhappy: they wished to have another child, and if she had more treatment and delayed the pregnancy, the child would not be born until the year of the chicken, which was unacceptable to them! We agreed to discuss it again at her next visit. And, finally, I saw Jeanne Perkins, whom I described previously in "Deja Vu." Her treatment had been complicated by severe allergic reactions to her basic medications, requiring me to "hyposensitize" her to the drugs: I restarted her medicines—one at a time—in literally miniscule doses. I hadn't utilized this procedure, for which the evidence of success was poor and the mechanism not well understood, in decades; nevertheless, the results were successful. Now her private physicians—a pulmonary doctor, an infectious disease specialist, her internist and her rheumatologist—all wanted to stop her TB medicines, even though she was continuing on her immune-destroying drug, and they asked for my assent. I could not and did not give it. What a clinic!

An Unshakeable Conviction

I was called by my clinic nurse to come to her office to review an x-ray on a new case of tuberculosis. Zhon Dang, a thirty-five-year-old woman, had come from China five years ago. She claimed to have had a positive skin test then, but we had no details. Now she had applied to a local hospital for a job, and because of the positive skin test history, she had a chest x-ray taken, which was reported to be abnormal. When I reviewed her x-ray, I noted clear-cut infiltrate in the right upper lobe with some strandy streaks of air within it, suggestive of an air bronchogram (the significance of an air bronchogram is that it only occurs with disease in the lung, not in the pleura, and often means inflammatory disease). Its location was a bit more medial than the usual TB lesion, and to my surprise, it was not visible in the lateral view. But I knew it had to be TB. I asked for sputum, and I ordered chemotherapy to be started.

A couple of days later I had another call. The x-ray had been repeated and was now said to be negative. Her doctor had told her to stop treatment, but I asked that she continue until we saw her at the next regularly scheduled clinic. When she came, it was with her husband, also Chinese; he was said to have a medical degree, but he was working as a technician in Pathology.

I reviewed both sets of x-rays. The shadow, just a few days later, was clearly gone! What were the possibilities? Perhaps the films were of different patients? But looking at the bones and elsewhere this was clearly the same body. Perhaps she had had pneumonia, which had cleared up? This we could check by reviewing her symptoms, but they were non-existent. I was reminded of one other, somewhat unlikely, possibility: in the old days we sometimes saw women with long hair which had not been placed on top of their heads for the x-ray. This sometimes resulted in the hair masquerading as intrapulmonary shadows.

I went to see her and her husband. Sure enough, she had a striking long, single braid of hair hanging down to her mid back. She remembered that it had not been raised at the time of the first x-ray, but had been raised at the second. The original radiologist—and I—had fallen into an old trap! The failure of the technician to follow a basic routine by positioning her hair correctly had almost led to a serious outcome.

I reviewed her story. Yes, she had had a positive skin test upon immigration, but her private doctor had taken an x-ray, said it was normal, and had not treated her preventively.

But the question remained: Why had the second x-ray been taken in the first place? The husband responded. "I knew she did not have TB," he said, "because she had no symptoms." He was, of course, quite wrong. Tuberculosis is often asymptomatic until the advanced stages, and many persons have refused therapy because of the lack of symptoms, only to regret it later when the disease progressed.

There was no point in reviewing the issue with Zhon Dang's husband, nor did I even try. He had been absolutely right to have had the x-ray repeated, but for the entirely wrong reason. A little bit of knowledge can go the wrong way. Nevertheless, it is surely better for anyone to be right for the wrong reasons, than to be wrong; sadly, however, it makes it extremely difficult to deal with such a person. Mr. Dang could never ever be convinced that his reasoning was incorrect.

Tuberculosis was, and continues to be, a fascinating disorder, with a long, even romantic, history. I continued to be enlightened over the years by my experience with hundreds of TB patients as to the many ways the disease could manifest itself within the body. The complex interrelationships between germ, host, and society were even more engaging and important both for science and for the public health. Remarkably, hosts of physicians spent their entire professional lives dealing with just this single disease, and were not only satisfied but also never bored doing so. Syphilis was similar, before penicillin, but I doubt any other disorder could so satisfy, although recently HIV-AIDS seems comparable. Today tuberculosis is rarely a fatal disease in the Western world, but unfortunately, such is not the case in many developing countries. The disease is still prevalent among large third-world populations, and the resources to treat those infected are severely limited. The World Health Organization estimates nine million new cases each year and a million deaths. The problem is compounded with the negative impact tuberculosis and HIV-AIDS have on each other, and the apparent inability or unwillingness of some nations to attack this problem. It is my hope going forward that an alliance of private foundations, non-profit organizations, such as the American Lung Association, governments, and non-governmental units will lead to a happier outcome for future generations.

Ann Arbor

An Old Saw

I came to Ann Arbor in 1958 to join the faculty of the University of Michigan Medical School, with the position of Chief of the Tuberculosis division at its affiliated Veterans Administration Hospital. When I arrived in Michigan, numerous tuberculosis sanatoria still existed throughout the state. I was not acquainted with them, but assumed they varied in quality, as had been my experience elsewhere. I soon received a transfer from one of them: Carl Brown had previously had tuberculosis in his left lung. It had been arrested by bed rest; but now he had new disease in his right lung. The physicians at the sanatorium had not isolated the TB germ. Based on a Papanicolau smear of his sputum, they had diagnosed cancer.

I studied Brown's x-ray. To me the location of the new spots in the axillary portion of the right upper lobe strongly suggested a relapse of the left-sided tuberculosis, not an unusual occurrence in the days before effective chemotherapy. Our sputum exams for malignant cells were negative, and our pathologist could not confirm their presence in the material sent from the sanatorium.

I presented the case to my consultants. Unanimously they agreed that TB was likely, cancer not so.

How wrong we were. After our studies for TB proved negative, bronchoscopy revealed a small cancer in the bronchus to the right upper lobe: the only manifestation of its presence was the shadows distally in the lobe.

163

It was a wonderful, if humbling, feeling to discover we were wrong. It surprised me that we university physicians had erred, when the group at the sanatorium had presumably stumbled onto the correct diagnosis. With the arrogance of youth barely suppressed, I wrote what I hoped was a politically correct letter to the physicians there. I gave them the follow-up information, credited their acumen, and asked how they had done it. In his reply Dr. Al Kempter gave a number of scientific reasons how they had reached their diagnosis based on their experience; but then, in a hand-written postscript, he added, "Even a blind hog turns up an ear of corn every now and then."

It was my first Midwestern experience with that old saw (dare I say old *sow*?). Al and I later became good friends and often laughed about our shared experience.

When All Else Fails

One night I received a call at home a few weeks after I started working at the Ann Arbor VA. It was from Rosalie Ging, head of the Psychiatry service, requesting immediate transfer of a patient, Perry Elston, from her unit (where he had been admitted with senile dementia) to the TB ward. She had been reviewing some lab slips, and noted (late) that Mr. Elston, admitted in October, had been reported to have a hazy nodule in the right upper lobe; a repeat x-ray, for some reason, in December had suggested the nodule now had air in it, that it was a cavity, and thus, the patient was suspect for tuberculosis. Somewhat reluctantly, without a real consultation, I approved the transfer.

Upon admission to my ward by standard procedure the first year resident performed a history and physical, and then the next day presented the patient to me. I saw the x-ray with the shadows of the spot and the space within it. They were atypical, with no shadows of inflammation at all around them. I ordered a work-up with a TB skin test and sputum for TB and for malignant cells, though his secretions were minimal. Shortly thereafter, the house officer came to me saying that Mr. Elston had developed high fever, headache, sputum production and shortness of breath. He suggested some rare disease had spread all through Elston's lungs. I went to the bedside. I found an elderly man, sitting up on the edge of his bed, leaning forward and breathing hard. I quickly checked his back and listened to his lungs; he was full of the moist noises called rales. They signified heart failure—the "rare disease" the house officer had not recognized. Elston had purulent secretions from his nose, and it appeared that an acute sinusitis in this frail elderly man had tipped him over into heart failure. The x-ray, which indeed showed changes throughout, was also strongly suggestive of heart failure. I instructed the skeptical house officer how to treat him and left.

Later that week Mr. Elston had improved, but one of the sputum samples was positive for malignant cells. I was surprised: even if the nodule were malignant, it would be rare for so small a lesion to produce malignant cells in the sputum. I thought perhaps the increased secretions from the infection had raised a few cells that otherwise would not have been expectorated.

I went to Elston's bedside to examine him more carefully. Another old medical aphorism suggests that when all else fails, resort to the physical examination! I found Perry comfortably lying flat, as his heart failure had resolved. I removed his pajama top. And there, on the front of his right upper chest, was a large pedunculated mole. (Medically, it was probably a pigmented seborrheic keratosis.) It was attached only at its upper end, and the lower portion was mobile. Could this skin lesion be responsible for the x-ray shadow? It was easy to see how movement of the lower portion could have trapped air under it, and simulated a space within the shadow on the x-ray. How to prove it? I took Elston to the x-ray department and, after repeating the x-ray, I took a Q-tip, moistened it with the radio-opaque barium used in GI x-ray exams, painted the floppy skin tag with it, and retook the x-ray. Sure enough, the "pulmonary" nodule had now become quite dense—the cause of the shadow was not a lung lesion, but a skin lesion. I took a stunning color photo of his chest and used those x-rays and the photo for years to teach the point that cutaneous bumps can simulate lung shadows. I would ask my residents how a shadow could "calcify" in the space of a few hours!

With Perry, a problem still remained: the positive Papanicolau smear for malignant cells. When our superb cytologist was presented with the story, he withdrew his diagnosis. He had thought the cells were excessively bizarre; in retrospect, they probably represented some abnormal infected cells from the sinusitis. And so ends the complex story of Perry Elston!

Oh, No, They Can't Take That Away From Me

Chest physicians are always showing each other cases, starting with the chest x-ray, for fun, for interest, for education. A spirit of competition, nevertheless, underlies much of our behavior. This case fooled me, will it fool him? Will she see the unusual x-ray finding? Could he possibly figure this one out? And so it goes.

In such spirit, my colleagues presented a case to me at Chest conference, soon after my arrival in Ann Arbor. They told me the x-ray was that of a young woman from a nearby Michigan city. She had developed a mild cough and some shortness of breath. An x-ray revealed widespread lung shadows known as infiltrates. Multiple usual and unusual studies had been unrevealing; eventually an operative biopsy of her lung had been performed. The findings were abnormal, but exactly what the diagnosis was remained unclear. At that point she was referred to the University. This was the only information I was given, but I could tell by their looks that my colleagues thought they had determined the answer. Competitive flags were flying!

I looked at the two chest x-rays, which had been taken a few weeks apart before her biopsy. The abnormality appeared the same in both. The lungs were filled with multiple, small non-discrete and non-specific shadows. Unfortunately, literally hundreds of conditions could cause this. Any one of them could be responsible, and I saw no clues on the x-ray or in the short history I was given, to lead me in one direction or another.

A tricky one—how to proceed? I decided to follow one of the principles I have always taught my students: "look all over," examine every inch of the x-ray, top to bottom, side to side. I did, and still, nothing stood out. But then, at the top of the first x-ray, I noticed that the woman's long hair, which hung down to her shoulders, had multiple hairpins in it. In the second x-ray, the hairpins were replaced by half a dozen curlers. Her hair appeared to be of great importance to her. Aha! A condition had recently been described in which women who used hair spray excessively had breathed much of it into their lungs; the lungs reacted and an abnormal condition much like this developed. The condition had been termed "thesaurosis." The word, "thesaurus," refers to treasure, the lungs being viewed as a treasure chest for the abnormal material. Triumphantly pointing out these clues, I concluded that this was a case of thesaurosis!

The looks on my colleagues' faces indicated I must be correct. In taking her history carefully, they had found she was a professional hair dresser, who was exposed daily to excessive amounts of hair spray. When they had raised the possibility with our pathologist, who reviewed the biopsy material from the other hospital, he had concurred.

A brilliant diagnosis! Word of my perspicacity—my coup—spread rapidly. As a feather in my cap, it was a tale worth telling and retelling, and certainly, a case worth adding to the teaching file. But one minor problem developed: over the next few years pathologists and researchers reviewing the entire concept, and especially the abnormal tissue reaction, decided that, actually, such changes in the lung did not really indicate a new and different condition. Instead, they were compatible with a known disorder, sarcoidosis.

Now, sarcoidosis itself is a disease of unknown cause, or causes. Some believe we have simply not yet discovered its cause; but others think a change in the body's reactivity underlies the condition, and that many environmental substances may elicit a similar reaction, resulting in the presence of "sarcoid tissue" in the body. If so, thesaurosis would be a form of sarcoidosis, specifically caused by one or more ingredients in hair spray.

So, one school of thought attributes my patient's condition to the more common sarcoidosis. And in fact, if you look at many medical textbooks and reviews, you will find that they do not list thesaurosis anywhere among the unusual pulmonary disorders, nor do they list hair spray as a cause of any specific pulmonary disease. A second school of thought attributes my patient's condition to being a form of sarcoidosis, caused specifically by exposure to hair spray. Still a third school of thought, much in the minority, maintains that thesaurosis exists as its own distinct disorder.

What do I believe? *How can I give up my brilliant diagnosis*? What an irony, if they try to take it away from me by suggesting I had diagnosed a non-existent condition! I believe in thesaurosis; it would be another of life's great injustices if it did not exist.

Surely I am not the first, nor will I be the last, to have my ego affect my judgment. And by this I am comforted.

An Addictive Pattern

A resident presented the case to me, along with a group of students and house officers. The patient, Henry Hardy, had been admitted for generalized abdominal pain. The abnormal x-ray was a surprise, as his only chest complaint was a nonproductive cough. As the presentation continued, I studied the films. The man had numerous patchy and conglomerate shadows involving both lower lobes and the right middle lobe. I also looked through his thick x-ray jacket. In it I found many other films, including two prior barium enemas, suggesting either chronic or recurrent bowel problems. By the time the presentation concluded, I had come to a conclusion beyond that of a mere educated guess. It was still early in my career at Ann Arbor; I wished to impress the residents as a means of increasing interest in lung disease, and perhaps, to start a fellowship program. I decided to show off a bit. I said, "We will go to the bedside and talk to Mr. Hardy. I will ask him how are his bowels, and he will tell us he suffers from constipation. I will ask what he takes for it, and he will say mineral oil. And when I ask if he takes a teaspoon or tablespoon, he will smile shyly and say that he actually drinks it directly from the bottle."

Of course, that is exactly what happened, except for the shy smile.

Constipation, with or without accompanying hemorrhoids, was, and is, a frequent problem. Mineral oil has long been an effective remedy for it and other painful anal conditions. It was heavily used, particularly in nursing homes and for neurologic patients, but usage was by no means limited to them. The advent of stool softeners has reduced the consumption of mineral oil markedly, but it is still popular. It is not commonly aspirated into the lungs when taken by the spoonful, but many persons found a swig from the bottle easier. With the head thrown back, the smooth and non-irritating material could easily slip into the lungs where over time, it stimulated inflammation and scarring. The changes, medically termed "lipoid pneumonia," often went undiscovered until a routine chest x-ray was taken.

Hardy was advised of the diagnosis. We recommended he use other means to relieve his constipation. Whether he did or not, I do not know. What I do know is that many patients find mineral oil so helpful that they become, as it were, addicted to it.

A few years later, my first pulmonary fellow who had been present during Hardy's presentation, brought me a fascinating consultation from the Neurology service. Roy Newhouse had an unusual anomaly of his cervical spine; it was also suspected that he had syringomyelia, a destructive disorder of the cervical spinal cord. In any case, he was partially paralyzed. Still in his twenties, he was diligently cared for at home by his mother, but a recent exacerbation had led to his hospitalization.

His chest x-ray revealed streaky densities in both of his mid-lung fields extending out from the center. In the lateral view these were located far back in the upper portions, the superior segments, of his lower lobes. The residents and I discussed the possibilities. I suggested, in a neurologic patient, lipoid pneumonia. But the location, said my fellow, is atypical. I agreed. We went to the bedside, finding his mother there, and Roy in his wheel chair. It did not take long to confirm the use of mineral oil. "Could you tell us how you give it to him?"

"Well, actually, it is the last thing I do for him at night. I help him into bed and then, while he is lying down on his back, I give him a tablespoonful of mineral oil." The position was exactly that which would permit the oil to flow into the upper portions of the lower lobe, rather than at the bases, as it did in those who were upright. We told Mrs. Newhouse about what had happened and recommended she discontinue use of the oil.

A decade later I worked in the Dean's office of the medical school, spending only a small portion of my time at the VA Hospital. One day a former fellow, who was now Chief of the Division, told me he wished to show me a remarkable case. He put up the x-ray; it showed immense widespread changes throughout the lungs accompanied by an enlarged heart, a situation in which extensive lung disease had led to heart failure. But, in the neck, I noticed a telltale abnormality of the cervical spine. "Is the man's name Roy Newhouse?" I asked. My colleague was surprised as indeed it was. Whether his mother had temporarily discontinued using mineral oil or not, we did not know, but it was obvious that she had later resumed its use. Clearly in her mind, its positive effect outweighed any negative concerns, eventually to the tragic detriment of her son.

One would hope stool softeners will eventually eliminate the use of mineral oil as a laxative.

The Look

John Oriskany was fifty-two when he was transferred to our hospital. He had been in and out of an excellent community hospital for three months, suffering from recurrent episodes of high temperature without localizing symptoms or physical findings. His records came with him. He was anemic; his white blood count was elevated; he had a minor non-specific abnormality on his electrocardiogram, but the multiple additional studies had all failed to determine the cause of his febrile illness. Fever of unknown origin was, and is, a frequent diagnostic problem, and Oriskany's problem was typical. Many reported series of cases of the syndrome have revealed that three categories of illness are responsible for the majority: infections, cancers, and disorders of the connective and vascular tissues.

Initial studies in our hospital were also nonspecific, and a connective tissue disorder, difficult to diagnose in 1961, was suspected. I was asked to see Oriskany, because of a minor abnormality on his chest x-ray: his left diaphragmatic leaflet, normally smooth and curved, was slightly straightened and irregular. I went to his bedside. He lay stiffly in bed, on his left side, covers up to his neck, his skin warm to the touch. And then there was his face: deep set eyes, pinched dry lips, mouth slightly open, cheeks drawn and flushed red. I knew that look. And so did other medical men back to Hippocrates, the legendary Greek physician of the 5th century BCE—in fact, the look, termed the "Hippocratic facies," was named after him. Hippocrates said it was a sign of peritonitis, inflammation of the lining of the abdomen; although it can be seen after a prolonged and wasting illness, most modern physicians have found no reason to disagree.

In 1961 I still had a fluoroscopic unit adjacent to my tuberculosis ward. I took Oriskany there and, as suspected, his left diaphragmatic leaflet moved minimally as compared to the right. I made my diagnosis, a difficult and uncommon one, and recorded it: Left subdiaphragmmatic abscess; recommend surgical drainage. True, I could not explain why an abscess had developed, especially in this unusual location, but the few findings, plus the look, convinced me I was correct.

To my surprise and distress, the physicians responsible for his care were not shaken from their initial diagnosis; it took much discussion to convince his physicians to ask the surgeons to see Oriskany. But the surgeons, too, were unconvinced, suspecting a lymphoma as the cause of his fevers. What to do?

I reviewed my findings, considered multiple other possibilities, but concluded as I had originally. Recalling Betty Foster from my sanatorium days, I suggested I perform a pneumoperitoneum, a procedure in which air would be introduced into the peritoneal cavity. In the upright position the air would rise to the sub diaphragmatic spaces, but an abscess would have obliterated the space and prevented the rise on the left. (Today a CT scan of his abdomen would confirm or deny my diagnosis instantly, but the multiple radiologic studies of that earlier era were not diagnostic.)

Oriskany soon helped solve the problem. He began to cough up foul material, due either to a new pneumonia in his poorly ventilated left lower lobe, or to rupture of the abscess through the diaphragm. Now I

171

did perform the pneumoperitoneum and confirmed my diagnosis. The surgeons drained almost two liters of thick pus from his abdomen.

What was most remarkable to me was how, as he recovered, his face filled out and lost its flush. The look was gone!

Years later investigators at Michigan State University were studying the diagnostic process used by master clinicians. I was flattered to have been chosen to be one of their experts. I was presented with a number of situations, and my responses were taped for analysis. One such experiment involved a theoretical patient whose history suggested ulcerative colitis to me. When I asked for certain studies, the findings pointed instead to a liver illness. I went back and forth, checking and rechecking, but I could not reconcile or correlate the history with the other studies. I worried about it all the next week, but when I returned for my next session I was told that, by error, I had been given the findings for another patient! I told the investigators that they had a marvelous unplanned experiment on tape: how clinicians behave—checking and rechecking—in the presence of conflicting data. Sadly, to me, they did not include the case in their published book on the diagnostic process.

Eventually...

Elzia Jacobs, a sturdy large-boned working man and heavy smoker, was admitted to the general medical ward for an exacerbation of both cough and joint pains, mostly in the knees and ankles. He was diagnosed with rheumatoid arthritis, and treated for pneumonia in the left lower lobe. We were consulted. Don Stevenson, a handsome, bright, self-assured man, was my resident. We reviewed the case. Although Jacobs's breath sounds were not as prominent as I had expected, he had rales—those little crackling sounds—in his left lower lobe that betokened infection. His chart included record of a prior pneumonia on the right, with some bronchial damage demonstrated by a bronchogram, a procedure in which dye is inserted into the bronchial tree. When I took his history, I was impressed with the fact that each time he had an exacerbation of his pulmonary disease, he also appeared to have an exacerbation of his arthritis. I diagnosed his condition as recurrent pneumonia, complicated by hypertrophic pulmonary osteoarthropathy (HPO). The name is a mouthful. HPO is a rare bone and joint complication, usually associated with pulmonary malignancy; but I had seen a few patients in whom it had occurred with benign disease and felt certain this was the situation with Jacobs. He was discharged before further studies were done; the discharge diagnoses—ignoring my opinion—were stated as pneumonia and rheumatoid arthritis.

Jacobs was readmitted two months later with another exacerbation of both conditions. His left lower lobe disease had extended further with some destruction of the lung, and his breath was foul. Dr. Robinson, the Chairman of Internal Medicine, was rheumatology consultant at the time, and he saw Jacobs. Not surprisingly, he quickly realized the rheumatoid arthritis diagnosis was incorrect; this, he suggested, was HPO, agreeing with my previous diagnosis. X-rays of his bones and joints confirmed the changes one expects to see in HPO.

However, he also said that because Jacobs had HPO, the pulmonary diagnosis was lung cancer, instead of pneumonia. We were again consulted. Now, one did not casually disagree with Dr. Robinson, who was not only Chairman of the Department, but was also, deservedly, widely respected as an excellent physician and diagnostician. I reviewed the findings and the physical exam; I saw no reason to depart from my prior diagnosis of benign, rather than malignant, disease and stuck to my guns. I consented to further studies to clarify matters: Jacobs was bronchoscoped, and no tumor was found; nor was there any evidence of a tumor seen on another bronchogram. It did, however, demonstrate that he had a large lung abscess, which some thought must be malignant.

I instituted treatment of the abscess with postural drainage and high doses of antibiotics with only moderate success. Eventually we had to resect his entire left lower lobe, which did bring about a "cure" of that condition. A very careful dissection of the resected tissues showed no evidence of cancer. Jacobs no longer experienced the exacerbations of joint pain with respiratory infections. "But you wait," the skeptics said, "he will eventually turn out to have cancer."

I continued to see Jacobs in follow up for years, as he was an excellent teaching case. I would not say we became friends, but we were long-established acquaintances who greeted each other warmly on each visit. Then, twenty-two—twenty-two!—years later he developed a large mass in the remainder of his left lung, which did turn out to be an inoperable lung cancer. It was not associated with a recurrence of his joint problems. He received chemotherapy, but eventually succumbed to his illness.

I dare say there still may be some who believe their earlier predictions of Jacobs "eventually" having cancer were correct. But in my mind there is no doubt, despite the rarity of the association, that the HPO was associated with his benign disease, rather than the cancer of twenty-two years later. To me Jacobs exemplifies the singularity of each patient, and the continuing importance of the history and physical examination in diagnosis. We teach students that "if you hear hoofbeats think of horses, not zebras;" but I always add that "if you see an equine animal with stripes, it is more likely to be a zebra than a horse in striped pajamas."

You Explain It

Richard King was thirty-four, a hardworking young man—a meat cutter—with a wife and three small children. For a couple of months it seemed he would get a chest cold that would pass off and then recur every two weeks or so; finally, an x-ray was taken which showed disease, including a cavity, in his right upper lobe, with some scattered spots in his left lung. There was not much question about the diagnosis: with his history and age and with this x-ray appearance, he obviously had tuberculosis. King was quickly admitted to the State Tuberculosis Sanatorium in Howell, Michigan.

Anti-TB medications were started promptly, but his physicians were in for a few surprises. His sputum did not reveal TB germs; in fact, his skin test for tuberculosis was also negative. In those days skin tests for a fungus disease common to this area—histoplasmosis—were popular, and King's test was positive. And yet further tests for that organism were also negative. Bronchoscopy, in which a lighted tube was passed through the vocal cords to inspect the bronchial tubes, was done twice, and both tests were inconclusive. Now after a few weeks and fair certainty the diagnosis was not tuberculosis, King was transferred to the Veterans Hospital in Ann Arbor.

Here a third bronchoscopy was more revealing. What appeared to be a tumor mass projected from the orifice of the right upper lobe and specimens taken from it were suspicious for cancer. King had been a heavy smoker since his teens, and despite his young age, cancer was a plausible diagnosis. He was taken to the operating room. Once more, his physicians were in for a surprise.

The anatomy of the bronchial tubes is such that the right upper lobe comes off the main bronchus to the right lung very close to the dividing line, called the carina, between the two lungs. To remove the tumor, removal of the entire right lung, a pneumonectomy, was necessary. But—in addition, a large fist-sized mass of cancerous lymph nodes was found in the mediastinum, the compartment that separates the two lungs. The mass even compressed the superior vena cava, the major vein carrying blood from the upper half of the body back to the heart. The surgeon described actually "scraping" the tumor off that vital vein to remove this mediastinal mass.

But the surprises were not over: the pathologist found the mediastinal mass to be all cancer; the edge, the margin of the removed bronchus showed tumor there as well, indicating tumor had clearly been left behind. The cell type was the most malignant of all, the "oat cell" variety of lung cancer. If any of these anatomic or cell type facts had been known preoperatively, surgery would not have been performed; as the cancer was incurable, there would have been no point to it.

Most of King's physicians were therapeutically aggressive, but their notes in the chart clearly indicated the surgical removal had been "subto-tal" and only "palliative;" radiation treatments would probably be futile, but could be given if and when the need developed. (Today chemotherapy is very effective, albeit temporarily, for this form of lung cancer, now known as undifferentiated small-cell cancer; King's illness occurred long before this era.) Richard was discharged to spend what little time he had left with his family, who were told he had only a short time to live.

I had not yet come to the VA when these events occurred. But *three full years later* I was there when King was transferred from another hospital with what appeared to be pneumonia in his remaining lung. I continued vigorous treatment for it and then, with resultant total incredulity, I reviewed his chart and x-rays. The left-sided spots seen originally had calcified, and they had surely represented histoplasmosis, rather than tumor. But something had to be wrong: survival like this from an untreated oat cell cancer was unheard of. Obviously, the pathologist must have erred three years earlier. Perhaps this had been a lymphoma, or even an inflammatory condition. I called to have the slides reviewed, and studied them myself with the pathologist. It was extraordinarily clear that there had been no error: this was about the best example of an oat cell cancer one could find. Had he received radiation (or some early form of chemotherapy), there was absolutely no doubt his survival would have been attributed to that treatment.

As King's pneumonia improved we subjected him to multiple tests, but could find no evidence of residual or recurrent cancer. I presented his case to a group of specialist consultants from the University. They all felt that, although his disease might yet recur, this was a rather incredible case—as the operative notes confirmed that complete removal of the tumor had simply not been possible.

So how could it have happened? Perhaps, I postulated, his massive tumor load had elicited some kind of antibody response, no matter how meager or ineffectual. Then, with the removal of the tumor, those antibodies had been able to contain the presumably small amounts of residual tumor.

I followed Richard regularly in my clinic, and came to know him and his family reasonably well. Then, after five years, I wondered whether or not I should pronounce him "cured." He was again presented to a group of consultants who were willing, tentatively, to call him cured. They felt his status was not a surgical cure, but that it probably reflected spontaneous regression of his tumor; thus, surgery for similar cases was not warranted. No new thoughts were offered about possible mechanisms for his survival.

Two years later, seven years after King's initial surgery, he developed high blood pressure. His chest x-ray remained stable, though his windpipe—the trachea—which had shifted to the right because that lung had been removed, seemed to have moved back towards the mid line. We could find no evidence for an elevated BP in his prior records. He might have had essential hypertension, that is, hypertension of unknown cause, but we felt it was important to study him for some curable form. Our initial studies were negative; in order to examine the blood vessels leading to the kidney, the procedure at that time, long since obsolete, was to inject dye directly into the aorta through the back. Unfortunately his sole remaining left lung was punctured by the procedure; it was promptly re-expanded, but despite that, King developed multiple pulmonary, cardiac and cerebral complications. It was as if his body had just fallen apart. A month later he died.

At autopsy we found no special explanation for the high blood pressure. The final surprise—at least to most of us—was that King was simply full of tumor, from his neck to his pelvis, filling the mid line spaces of his body. Microscopic slides showed the same malignant oat cell tumor as the material of seven years previously.

I talked to Mrs. King, whom I now knew fairly well, afterwards. I told her about the findings, and once again said how remarkable and unusual his course had been, and that we had no rational explanation for it. And Mrs. King said, "Well, he was so young when he first became ill. I think God gave him those seven years so he could watch, and help, his boys grow up." I replied that probably was as good an explanation as any.

Working with the theory that King's blood might contain anti-cancer antibodies, I had earlier taken some of his blood, pipetted off the serum, and frozen it in the laboratory. I thought that someday, perhaps, we would be able to study it for the antibodies or other substances that could have influenced his course. Some years later after a power failure, someone cleaned out the freezers; King's tubes were discarded.

Richard King is a medical "teaching case," one I would like all physicians, all oncologists, all biologists to know about. Why? Because I believe he exemplifies the variability that is inherent in all biology. The hardest task physicians have is prognosis, the prediction of outcome. We develop bell shaped curves, averages for survival, statistical methods to predict what may happen, concepts regarding the natural history of disease, statistical findings about treatment. Recently, the term "outliers" has been created to suggest that oh yes, there may be a case now and then that doesn't fit our algorithms. I do not like the term. It suggests our data on averages are correct, even if some don't fit the mold. I would rather the concept of inherent biological variability, as exemplified by Richard King, was better accepted and understood.

My Face is My Fortune

Ken Jackson was a Civic Theater stalwart in the 1960s and '70s. He was a funny-looking guy with gargoylish features who, for example, played a non-speaking butler in *Major Barbara* and stole every scene he was in. He and I had known each other for years. I was a popular faculty member among the Internal Medicine residents, and I had talked about Civic Theater to them. *Guys and Dolls* was running; Ken played Harry the Horse, perhaps an example of type casting. A group of the residents, including one named Newell Augur, came to see the show. I sat in the orchestra, while they were all up in the balcony. After the show, they come down to tell me how much they had enjoyed it. "And," said Newell, "that acromegalic was terrific!" What?! and Wow!!

Acromegaly is a disease in which the pituitary gland becomes overactive because of hyperfunction or a tumor. If the disease starts in childhood, it results in gigantism—great height and very long extremities; if in adulthood, the hands and feet and facial bones enlarge grotesquely. The changes are characteristically very, very slow, so gradual that family and friends often do not recognize there is anything wrong, unless old photographs are studied. Ken's case was typical. I had not recognized the change, whereas smart observant medical residents were able to make the diagnosis from the balcony of the Lydia Mendelssohn Theater!

Ken entered the hospital, and the diagnosis was established. He was told that he should be treated with radiation therapy or surgery to stop the growth of the probable pituitary tumor. His facial features might regress slightly towards normal. As he had no other symptoms, treatment was not mandatory, but he would have to watch carefully for new ones, such as headache and visual difficulties. Ken thought about it, but then said, "My face is my fortune." He declined treatment. He went to Hollywood and did, indeed, make a living from his face. You have seen him as a truck driver in numerous commercials, and in small bits in many films. In "Forget Paris," the camera focuses on him as an irate and raucous fan. He eventually did receive treatment.

My colleague Ralph Knopf is the endocrinologist who took care of Ken here. When he tells the story, he often credits me with the diagnosis. It is a much better medical story that I missed, rather than made, the diagnosis, because that is both the truth of the story and characteristic of the disorder.

George Jones and the Mikado

George Jones was a pretty routine case for those days, the sixties. He had had trouble with an ulcer—a duodenal ulcer—for years, and was in the hospital for surgery on his stomach to correct the situation. The surgery went well. At its completion, however, as the anesthesiologist removed the intratracheal tube—the tube down the windpipe which had permitted him to control George's breathing during the surgery and suction the secretions—he noted, to his surprise, some stomach contents within the trachea. Somehow, during the procedure, some vomitus or regurgitation had slipped past the tube. This aspiration of acidic fluid into the lung could be dangerous and could cause inflammation and destruction of the lung. And, in fact, an x-ray taken after the operation did show some shadows in the right lower lobe, far in the back in what is called the superior segment, the commonest location for this sort of problem. The surgeons treated him with an antibiotic, ordered him to start getting out of bed earlier than usual, and encouraged him to cough. To their surprise, a few days later, the x-ray was worse, and continued to get worse, now showing some destruction of the lung called a cavity, an actual hole in the lung. Now postural drainage was ordered. In this procedure the patient is

179

placed in a position so that the diseased area is above the draining bronchus, thereby allowing gravity to help the fluid in the destroyed area be expelled. They also ordered private nurses to be with him twenty-fours a day to both tend to him and ensure the postural drainage orders were carried out. But all to no avail. A few days later Jones's condition was worse still, with a large cavity in the lung containing an air-fluid level, the fluid being pus which had collected in the space. It was a Friday when two interventions were scheduled: a consultation with me and my service to see if we could offer any help, and surgery to drain the abscess. The surgery was scheduled for Tuesday, the surgeons' next operating day.

When I reviewed the case I found no fault with the management as ordered. Nevertheless the x-rays showed the treatment had failed. It was clear his lung was not draining, but not clear why. Perhaps there was something obstructing the bronchus and keeping it from draining, or perhaps treatment was not being carried out effectively. With my team I went to his bedside. George Jones was in bed lying absolutely flat on his back, in just the position he should not have been. His nurse was sitting at the bedside. She was a young, chubby, red-cheeked, cheerful woman. "You are performing postural drainage?" I asked.

"Oh yes, doctor, every four hours, just as ordered," she said.

I then said, "Describe it to me."

She smiled. "Well, doctor, to tell you the truth, every time I even just sit him up, this terrible green stinking stuff comes out of his mouth. It makes him sick, and it makes me sick, so I just lay him back down again."

In *The Mikado*, by Gilbert and Sullivan, the Mikado orders an execution to take place. Koko, the executioner, describes the death of Nanki Poo, the heir to the throne—but then Nanki Poo shows up. Koko explains that in Japan the Mikado's word is law, so when the Mikado orders someone to be killed, he is as good as dead, and if he is as good as dead, why not just say so! The explanation is satisfactory, and the play ends happily. Not so in medicine. Doctors too often assume that because they have given, or written, or left an order, it is as good as carried out—but, as in this case, such an assumption is not always correct and can be dangerous for the patient.

I should add that, at that moment in Jones's hospital room, I felt like ordering an execution for that cheery, rather ineffectual, nurse.

What happened to George Jones? As it was clear any routine measures might well not be followed out, I ordered him placed in a Stryker frame. This device is a frame which can be rotated with the patient sandwiched between two canvas cots. George was kept in a face down position for long periods, being turned into other positions at intervals for comfort. He drained copiously. I saw to it that his x-ray was repeated on Monday afternoon, after fewer than 72 hours, and my expectation was fulfilled: to my pleasure the cavity had emptied of pus and reduced in size by fifty percent! With continued use of the frame, appropriate antibiotics and physical therapy, the surgical procedure proved unnecessary.

Unexpected Consequences

I'll call him Harry Lasser. He was an eighteen-year-old Michigan kid who, like so many others, was inducted into the Army at the height of the draft early in World War II. Harry was different, though. During induction he behaved peculiarly, and went off the deep end as soon as he arrived at a basic training camp. Sent to a military hospital for evaluation, he was diagnosed as schizophrenic, clearly unfit for service, and discharged. The process took ninety-two days, and the rule in those days was that after ninety days of service you became a veteran, eligible for veterans' benefits. So Harry was hospitalized at government expense at the Battle Creek Veterans Hospital, primarily a psychiatric hospital, during the forties, the fifties, and into the sixties.

Psychiatric care changed from simple warehousing during Harry's hospitalization. When medications became available, Harry received them. His erratic, wild behavior calmed down, and he became rather placid. He didn't do much, except eat and smoke and become fat. One of the common side effects of the drugs, tardive dyskinesia, affected Harry seriously. This condition consists of uncontrollable muscular movements, lack of coordination, and a peculiar protrusion and rolling of the tongue.

When the movement to empty psychiatric hospitals gained popularity, Harry was among those who were discharged. A foster home was found for him on a poultry farm in southern Michigan. It was a major change for Harry, who hadn't been out of the hospital for decades. He didn't do much on the farm, except sit on the porch and wander around, but he was outside much more than he had been. But the new environment—as sheltered as it was—was too much for him, and after six months he was returned to the Hospital. In one sense, this is where the story begins.

Upon readmission, Harry had a chest x-ray taken, and lo and behold, it was abnormal. A rounded density was visible in the left upper lobe, a new shadow that had not been there on the last x-ray Harry had had as an inpatient. Maybe it was pneumonia, as Harry had recently developed a slight cough. The x-ray was repeated a few weeks later: the shadow had enlarged and was now considered suspicious for tumor.

When I first arrived in Michigan, tuberculosis was common at Battle Creek, as it was at other mental hospitals. After seeing a number of patients transferred from there, many having been poorly handled, I visited the hospital, did some teaching for their staff, and established a regular quarterly conference at which I saw problem cases. (Battle Creek, like many residential psychiatric hospitals, was isolated on a large piece of property, and it had its own private golf course. My residents loved to go there with me. We would play golf in the morning and hold our conference in the afternoon.) Later, when problem cases were fewer, referrals were sent directly to me in Ann Arbor. Over the years, however, staffs changed, and our arrangement fell apart. When Harry's problem developed, his case was referred directly to the surgeons at our hospital.

A bit about surgeons from this internist's perspective: some surgeons consider themselves internists *plus*; that is, they do everything internists do, plus they operate. I have always disliked this attitude, because it implies that the time available to internists when NOT in the operating room is not important. On the contrary, the skills developed studying patients outside the operating room are different from and complementary to a surgeon's skills, and in some aspects may surpass them. In addition, surgeons naturally have a propensity to recommend surgery and feel that internists are too reluctant to consider the same; whereas, internists feel surgeons are often too quick to do so. Two phrases come to mind: *you never ask your barber if you need a haircut*; and one I heard first from Dr. Cameron Haight, a famed Michigan thoracic surgeon, *one peek is worth two finesses*. Both, of course, illustrate the surgeon's desire to operate and "explore."

Back to Harry. Our surgeons tentatively diagnosed cancer, ordered special x-rays called laminograms (the forerunners of CT scans), and admitted Harry to the hospital. As both a courtesy and a desire to exclude the possibility of tuberculosis, they sent a consultation to us, the internists.

When we saw Harry, the most remarkable thing about him was the tongue rolling; a fat man, he had not lost weight, but that by no means excluded cancer, especially with his smoking history. We studied the x-rays and the laminograms. We noticed there was not just one spot, but actually a few close together, some mass-like, some more patchy. In addition, the film on admission to our hospital looked better, as if the disease had begun to resolve, as compared to those x-rays taken when he first returned to Battle Creek. Our skin test for tuberculosis was negative. We strongly advised against surgery, feeling it was unnecessary. We suggested this was an inflammatory, not a neoplastic condition, although without further study we did not offer a specific alternate diagnosis. Instead of a resection, only a biopsy was performed.

In mystery cases like this, the secret is often in whatever is unique or unusual in the history or presentation. Can you guess what the key was?

Harry Lasser's case is a marvelous example of unexpected consequences. In the biopsy specimen, the pathologist found multiple areas of inflammation and reaction in the tissue, and special stains revealed the offending organism to be *Histoplasma capsulatum*—a fungus organism which grows in the soil, particularly in areas where the soil is fertilized by bird droppings. Humans contract histoplasmosis by breathing in dusty soil containing the organism. Harry Lasser, institutionalized for years, had been sent out of the hospital to a presumably peaceful and relaxing chicken farm in the hopes of a better life. Not only had he not been able to tolerate it, but he had also been exposed to this fungus, which led to hospitalization and multiple procedures. Sometimes the best intentions can result in the most peculiar and unexpected consequences.

Serendipity

Mr. Campbell was admitted to my service because he had an abnormal chest x-ray. That, however, seemed to be the least of it. A man in his sixties, his major difficulty was that he was blind. His loss of vision had come on gradually, beginning ten to fifteen years ago, and the cause had never been established. He had had a long sojourn at the Mayo Clinic where, he said, other than learning his blindness was permanent, he had not been helped.

Over the years he had become weaker and less able to care for himself; he had, thus, come to our hospital. His chest x-ray had a surprising finding: the upper lobe of his right lung was dense and shrunken towards the top of the right chest and the midline. Tuberculosis, fungal disease, or a tumor were all possibilities. Nothing special was noted on his physical examination other than obesity, a puffy face and slightly swollen ankles. As part of his workup, an intravenous pyelogram was ordered. In this procedure dye which is concentrated by the kidneys is injected into an arm vein. In contrast to the standard procedure, an x-ray was taken promptly after the injection for purposes of a research study; we found that the superior vena cava, the major vein that returns blood from the entire upper body to the heart, was blocked. And lo and behold, there we saw a fabulous picture, better than any anatomic dissection or drawing could ever illustrate: zillions of collateral veins demonstrating the myriad possibilities by which the venous system can adjust to the blockage of the cava and still get the blood back to the heart.

So, inadvertently, we made a diagnosis of superior caval syndrome in Mr. Campbell. Records from Mayo suggested it had probably been present then. The commonest cause of this situation is a tumor, but this was unlikely given his long-term history. We diagnosed a rare condition known as fibrosing mediastinitis, in which, for no known reason, scarring affects the tissues in the mediastinum (the space in the chest between the two lungs) and seriously obstructs the veins, and often, other structures as well. In Campbell's unusual case, the scarring had also invaded the right upper lung. We felt that, somehow, the blindness was also probably related. Unfortunately, there was not much we could do about this

184

condition, other than offer reassurance that a tumor was not involved, and that any progression would be as slow as it had been in the past.

Another serendipitous case is that of Jack Manchester. He had cirrhosis of the liver with massive collections of fluid in his abdomen (ascites) and feet. The elevated diaphragm compressed his lungs, and shadows—presumably due to the compression—were present in both lower lungs, more so on the left side. He was treated with diuretics to attempt to reduce the excess fluid and became mentally obtunded, perhaps because of resultant low blood volume or a chemical imbalance. As was standard, blood chemistries were therefore ordered. In those days each substance to be measured by the blood test had to be ordered individually, and on the lab order form the consecutive boxes for sodium, potassium, chloride and CO_2 each had to be checked. The box below CO_2 was for calcium; when the ward clerk carelessly checked four boxes in a row, she checked calcium instead of sodium. Surprise: the test result revealed that Jack's blood level of calcium was markedly elevated. This finding was, of course, totally independent of dietary intake. The causes of hypercalcemia are limited; one of the major ones is cancer. The high level was the serendipitous first tip off that the left sided lung disease was due to cancer, rather than simple compressed lung.

Samarra

Arthur McDonough was in his seventies when he was referred to our hospital for evaluation. He had two problems: the most pressing to public health authorities was the possibility of active tuberculosis; the second, of more concern to him, was his chronic lung disease.

The story we obtained from him was that, as many World War I veterans claimed, he had been "gassed" on the front lines in France. After the war ended, while still in uniform, tuberculosis had been diagnosed. He had been sent to a tent hospital for rest. Shortly after admission there, the Spanish influenza epidemic engulfed his hospital. Horrified by the dead and dying around him, McDonough had absconded, leaving the hospital without permission against the advice of his doctors.

The influenza epidemic of 1918-19 was one of the most serious plagues ever to affect man. It was a true pandemic, a worldwide catastrophe, killing more people, by far, than the war itself had. It left those who had lived through it, including McDonough, in mortal fear of a possible recurrence. He associated the risk with hospitalization; close contact with others, anywhere, was a more general concern.

Others who had never had influenza wondered if it was nothing more than a severe common cold. In 1945, I learned they were wrong. That winter an epidemic of influenza hit the country, and I was one of those who caught it. It was clear to me that the prostration, the general feeling of sickness and especially the severe muscle aches were quite different from symptoms of the common cold. Fortunately the flu that season was not particularly severe or life threatening, except in the elderly and those with diminished resistance to any illness.

Eleven years later, in 1956-7, I was on the staff of the Bronx VA Hospital when the Asian flu—named so, because it was believed to have originated in Asia and spread worldwide from there—hit the United States. The illness was much more serious than the 1945 variety, sometimes fatal in itself, and often complicated by fatal superinfection with bacteria, especially the staphylococcus. I learned much about it, including the suggestion that severe forms of the disease appeared to run in cycles of eleven years.

Now back to Mr. McDonough. After the war his wheezing and chronic cough persisted. He had reluctantly accepted a few short admissions to tuberculosis facilities for evaluation, but he believed nothing definitive had been established. In the 1960's one laboratory had claimed to have isolated the TB germ, and this prompted his admission to the VA.

We reviewed his x-rays. They did, indeed, show changes in the left upper lung, strongly suggestive of tuberculosis. However, these had not changed over a period of time. We thought it most likely that his disease had healed and was not active. To be certain, our routine was to collect sputum and examine it for the TB germ, both by looking for it under the microscope and by attempting to grow it in the laboratory. Meanwhile, it was clear that he did have some generalized pulmonary difficulty, which had resulted in shortness of breath and wheezing. McDonough, like most veterans, was a smoker. Differentiating the cause of his chronic bronchitis and emphysema—whether from the damage resulting from toxic gas exposure years ago, or from his heavy smoking—was moot. We scheduled tests of his pulmonary function since, regardless of cause, they were necessary to establish the degree of his disability.

And then our hospital, including our ward, experienced the 1967-8 Hong Kong influenza outbreak. McDonough, despite his assignment to a private room, caught the infection. It affected him severely, leading to pneumonia and heart failure, as was not rare for the elderly. Despite our attempts with the best we could offer in supportive care, McDonough succumbed. The cause of death was influenza, the illness he had feared and tried to escape in 1919.

John O'Hara introduces his novel *Appointment in Samarra* with this excerpt entitled "Death Speaks" by W. Somerset Maugham.

There was a merchant in Bagdad who sent his servant to market to buy provisions and in a little while the servant came back, white and trembling, and said, Master, just now when I was in the market-place I was jostled by a woman in the crowd and when I turned I saw it was Death that jostled me. She looked at me and made a threatening gesture; now, lend me your horse, and I will ride away from this city and avoid my fate. I will go to Samarra and there Death will not find me. The merchant lent him his horse, and the servant mounted it, and he dug his spurs in its flanks and as fast as the horse could gallop he went. Then the merchant went down to the market-place and he saw me standing in the crowd and he came to me and said, Why did you make a threatening gesture to my servant when you saw him this morning? That was not a threatening gesture, I said, it was only a start of surprise. I was astonished to see him in Bagdad, for I had an appointment with him tonight in Samarra.

I wonder if McDonough was aware of the story.

You Blew It

Mr. Solvang was listed as a new appointment for me in Pulmonary Clinic. I introduced myself, as I always did, and asked what was the trouble? It was difficulty breathing. I questioned him further and pretty soon he said, "I had been coming here for years, but you blew it. You people said I had emphysema, so I then went to the Mayo Clinic, and they took a biopsy and told me I have fibrosis." I was surprised. This distinction is not difficult to recognize, or at least should not be. At one point Solvang said that he thought he remembered me as being one of the mis-diagnosers! Now, of course, I was challenged. My immediate reaction was that he was wrong, particularly as he was listed as a new pulmonary patient. But his chart was a thick one, and so I commenced an exhausting search through it. It did not take me long to note that he had not been seen at our hospital for some years, but prior to that he had been a patient in the general medicine clinics. Dr. Noble had been his physician, and indeed his medications had been those prescribed for someone diagnosed with emphysema. I searched further. I finally found what I was looking for.

About ten years previously Dr. Noble, puzzled by this patient, or needing help, had consulted with us. Sure enough, it was I who had seen Solvang in consultation. I had noted a peculiar personality along with an underlying hostility, making it difficult to obtain a clear history. He was a member of Jehovah's Witnesses, and indeed the biopsy at Mayo Clinic had been of some concern, as it was done with the prohibition that blood be used, even if necessary. In any case, my notes had indicated his complaint to be shortness of breath, particularly on exertion, but I had found no explanation for it, even with a routine chest x-ray which had appeared entirely normal. On physical examination I found nothing to indicate any obstructive lung disease. Even his screening spirometric pulmonary function tests had been within normal limits. The only finding of note was during his physical exam when I heard a few rales at both bases posteriorly that should not have been there. They were widely scattered and not particularly impressive. I ended my consultation with my diagnosis: "This patient either has no disease, or very early interstitial

188

fibrosis." I offered suggestions for follow up and for further studies—suggestions that were basically ignored by Dr. Noble. Mr. Solvang had since been lost to our system for many years. Finally the recent biopsy at Mayo confirmed the diagnosis I had suspected years before.

I was proud that I had suspected the correct diagnosis at a very early stage, based primarily on the physical examination. I am only sorry that no further studies were implemented at that time when an early stage of fibrosis might have been more easily treated.

Captain Queeg

Would you ever have thought that Captain Queeg, the antihero of Herman Wouk's *The Caine Mutiny*, would make a positive contribution to my practice? Well, read on.

I began smoking cigarettes when I was seventeen. I became a regular smoker while in service, when a pack cost me $0.06 at the post exchange. It was the "smart" thing to do, and I enjoyed it. In the early 1950's, however, I became aware of the experimental work of Dr. Oscar Auerbach, with whom I had almost taken a residency position in pathology some years previously. His research, along with anecdotal evidence, some epidemiological studies, and my own clinical experience, convinced me of the causal relationship between smoking and lung cancer. After one personal attempt to stop failed because of the stress associated with the unexpected death of a close colleague, I successfully discontinued cigarette smoking when I was thirty. In addition, I began to recommend smoking cessation to my patients, both those with and without lung disease.

My recommendations were rarely followed. Few community supportive agencies were available then, and the public had not embraced the important concept of the serious danger of smoking. Cigarettes were easily purchased in hospitals and other health care facilities; many doctors continued to smoke; they, along with entertainment celebrities and political figures, were prominently featured in cigarette advertisements. Thankfully, times have changed!

As I continued to recommend cessation, however, I noticed different patterns of the functions cigarettes apparently played in my patients', as well as my friends', lives. Most got a "kick," a stimulus, from smoking; some, a good feeling associated with relaxation. They clearly were responding to the chemical contents of the cigarettes, elements that we know today are addictive. Some, however, seemed to have a need to have something in their mouths at all times, and a dangling cigarette, sometimes not even lit, fulfilled this need. Still others seemed to find it necessary to be always doing something with their hands and, once again, fiddling with a cigarette, removing it from a pack, tapping it against the pack, taking it back and forth from their mouths, was an important aspect of the habit.

I tried to accompany my recommendations with awareness of individuals' behavior, especially when they seemed responsive to my suggestions or, preferably, when they, themselves, expressed a desire to stop. For the chemically dependent some aids were available even early on, although nowhere near as effective as the patches and gums we have today. For those whose mouths seemed to need a workout, I recommended sucking non-sweet astringent cough drops. These left the mouth with a distinct sensation of dryness, or burning, which satisfied some. But what to recommend for those with nervous hands?

In the novel *The Caine Mutiny* the anti-hero, Captain Queeg, memorably played by Humphrey Bogart in the subsequent film, would remove shiny steel balls from his pockets in moments of stress and rotate them in his hands. His action was viewed as a sign of obsessive weakness by those who observed him. It made a recommendation for my patients to use them laughable. However, one of my friends came from a family of four brothers who were emotionally close, though often geographically separated. He had distributed glossy black hematite stones to his brothers; each kept one in a pocket and, when they touched a stone, each man gained a feeling of closeness to the others. For those patients whose hands were constantly moving, I began to recommend shiny stones in lieu of steel balls, making light of the association by often saying, "Now, this will sound like Captain Queeg..." I did not have great success.

One colleague and friend, an anatomist whom I will call Ray, smoked heavily. We had served on committees together, where I had noticed his hands in ceaseless motion. One day, in an informal session, he expressed the wish to stop smoking and asked for my advice. His collar was open but, fortuitously, he was wearing a tie; the tie was held to his shirt by a clasp with a shiny stone on it. In Michigan we are fortunate to have a specific fossil, the Petoskey stone, easily found by walking along the shores of our northern lakes. When ground and polished they often show endless variations of attractive fossil structures, and are well known throughout the state. Ray was wearing this very stone in his tie clasp. I seized the moment: I recommended he keep two or three small Petoskey stones in his pocket, and when he felt the need, either put his hand in his pocket and feel them, or especially when alone, remove them a lâ Queeg to look at them, rotate them, play with them.

Ray became my greatest success. He not only succeeded in stopping smoking himself, but he also became an advocate for my method with others, among whom the success rate was surprisingly high. I believe the social acceptability of the Petoskey stone added to the specific success of this technique among Michigan patients. Ray left our University some years later, but when he and I would see each other at meetings or reunions, he never failed to take a few stones from his pocket, show them to me, and we would laugh.

Cry Wolf

I knew Frank Pieczorek for years. He smoked, he drank, he may well have taken drugs—and he suffered the ravages expected from such behavior. He was single, unemployed, with no permanent address. He said his occupation had been "farmer," but if you asked him details about his life on the farm, he responded with a sly smile and an irrelevant answer.

Frank was first admitted to our hospital for the complications of alcoholism, most prominent of which was chronic liver damage, diagnosed as early cirrhosis. With cirrhosis, the liver tissue is scarred resulting in a reorganization of its structure and poor function of what remains. Excess fat also invades the organ. However, with the combination of rest, a good diet, vitamin supplementation and abstinence from alcohol, his liver recovered, demonstrating the remarkable ability of that organ to regenerate.

I met Pieczorek during his second admission. A chronic cough was now more prominent and was associated with some shortness of breath on exertion. When I saw him in consultation, I saw the stereotypical cartoon image of a chronic alcoholic. He was grizzled, unshaven, unkempt, toothpick dangling from dry lips, a dry red tongue and teeth in terrible condition. Just as expected, his breath sounds were not as loud as they should have been when I listened to his lungs, and I could elicit some wheezing noises when he breathed out forcefully. He clearly had chronic bronchitis as a result of his smoking. The x-ray of his chest was compatible with my diagnosis, and tests of the function of his lungs further confirmed it. When I suggested he stop smoking, he took the toothpick out of his mouth just long enough to laugh at me.

Pieczorek's third admission was different. He had been admitted complaining of an acute attack of abdominal pain, located in the midline above his umbilicus. The pain was severe and required narcotics for relief. Studies established a third diagnosis, this one also associated with alcoholism: inflammation of his pancreas, a condition known to be recurrent and often characterized by severe pain. Indeed, over the next year Frank was readmitted on multiple occasions, each time receiving narcotics, each time with pancreatitis suspected, although not always confirmed. There arose suspicion that he may have merely been seeking the narcotics, and that some of his complaints may have been factitious.

On his next admission a new diagnosis was made. His cough had worsened and become productive with grayish phlegm occasionally streaked with blood. His x-ray did not reveal the cancer one might have suspected, but instead, showed varying changes, including cavities, in the upper zones of both lungs. These findings strongly suggested tuberculosis, another condition not uncommon with his lifestyle. Laboratory examination quickly confirmed the diagnosis. Frank was transferred, along with his meager belongings—including a supply of the omnipresent toothpicks—to my inpatient tuberculosis ward.

At this time, inpatient hospitalization was the norm, at least until the disease was shown to be under control by the absence of TB germs in the sputum (and confirmed by the failure to continue growing TB organisms in the lab). Today, after an initial short period of hospitalization during which treatment would be started and the patient's cooperation established, a patient would be discharged to prolonged therapy, which tuberculosis still requires, on an outpatient basis. But in Frank's case outpatient treatment would have most likely been fraught with difficulty because of his self-destructive lifestyle. In any case, he actually enjoyed being on our ward. He found the situation non-stressful, and his relations with other patients and staff were pleasurable. Under my supervision, his daily medical care was in the hands of younger house officers in training, who usually spent one or two months on my service. During each period Frank would ordinarily have one or two bouts of abdominal pain and would usually receive narcotics for them. However, with time, it became known among the house staff that Frank was notorious for drug-seeking behavior; indeed, an episode of abdominal pain was often treated without much in the way of further examination to confirm the diagnosis of pancreatitis. I made sure to instruct new house officers to be wary of Frank's contrived illnesses when we reviewed his case in my conference room. This room was lined with x-ray view boxes, and on the walls I had framed prints of multiple medical aphorisms—some original, some familiar, some less so. One, for example, was from William Harvey, who was the first to discover and realize that blood circulates: "How base a thing it is to receive instruction from others' findings without examining them oneself." For me, this underscored the responsibility of physicians to always examine a patient—and x-rays—themselves.

About six months after his transfer, Frank's tuberculous disease was not yet fully controlled. The pattern of his recurrent abdominal pain and its treatment had become pretty well established. Then a new house officer, an internal medicine resident named Dale Baker, started on my service. A serious, thoughtful young man, Baker was initially clued in to the story of Pieczorek's drug-seeking behavior. He was therefore not surprised when a few nights later, Frank complained of severe midline abdominal pain. But Baker, perhaps aware of the quote from Harvey, carefully examined Frank's abdomen. He found the expected apparent tenderness to his palpation, but he also found the abdominal muscles rather rigid, in spasm. Baker ordered x-rays of the abdomen and chest, in both supine and upright positions. Surprise! The upright chest x-ray showed free air within the abdomen under the diaphragmatic leaflets, those muscles which separate the belly from the chest. Free air signifies a perforated abdominal air containing organ, such as the stomach or duodenum, most frequently due to an ulcer, and represents an acute surgical emergency.

The surgeons promptly took Pieczorek to the operating room. As expected, a perforated viscus was found. It was the small intestine, however, not the stomach. The unexpected cause was found there too: a sharp toothpick—probably swallowed carelessly and without Frank's conscious knowledge. It had punctured the bowel, allowing air and the bowel contents to soil the peritoneal space. Had Baker not performed his careful examination, made the diagnosis, and had the surgical exploration not been carried out, Pieczorek might well have cried wolf once too often, this time with a fatal outcome.

Recall the principle, "Eternal vigilance is the price of liberty"? And so it is with medicine, as so well demonstrated by Dale Baker and Frank Pieczorek. One could argue that it also makes the case for a preference for flossing over toothpicks!

Spots and Old Films

I believe strongly that today the history and physical examination of the chest and chest imaging studies are not competitive, but rather, complementary. Early on both approaches had extreme proponents: some phthisiologists—tuberculosis physicians—wrongly doubted the sensitivity and usefulness of the x-ray. And a Boston radiologist was said to have a stethoscope displayed in a cabinet with the label "A medieval instrument formerly used in the diagnosis of chest disease."

During my years of practice numerous other valuable diagnostic modalities were developed: the Papanicoloau smear, flexible fiberoptic instruments, ventilation/perfusion scans and computerized tomography (CT or Cat scans), and fine needle biopsy, to name just a few. None, however, replaced sound medical judgment. Or, as I liked to teach my students, "There is No Substitute for Brains." To demonstrate this particular dictum, I would present a case in which each new diagnostic modality had been inappropriately used or incorrectly interpreted. But then, I would present the next aphorism "Brains are Good, but Old films are better," emphasizing that despite our "brains," prior x-rays have often proved us wrong.

The following two cases, out of countless possibilities, successfully illustrate this second principle.

Israel Jakowski was an elderly man admitted to the hospital for cataract surgery. In those days all admissions had chest x-rays taken, a practice no longer considered productive, cost efficient or reimbursable. Jakowski's x-ray was abnormal: in his left upper lobe two spots, both roughly one centimeter in size, were clearly visible. One was round, very dense and sharply marginated, suggesting a lesion that may well have been there for some time. The other spot, however, was not dense, without sharp margins, and seemed to be extending into the surrounding tissues.

I spoke to Jakowski, who had no pulmonary symptoms, and informed him of the abnormality. He was not concerned; he told me that about five years previously in another state at the time of a hernia repair, the same thing had happened; that is, he had been told he had a spot in his left lung. His skin test for TB had been positive, but other studies were normal, and he had been told not to worry about it. I suspected he was correct in the sense that the dense lesion had probably been there, but surely, I prided myself in thinking, I am smart enough to recognize the different character of the second shadow. "Mr. Jakowski," I said, "you now have two spots; one looks like it has been there for a while, but the other looks 'softer' and fresher, and I am afraid it probably represents an active condition, like tuberculosis." I did not mention the possibility of a tumor.

We ordered additional studies, meanwhile sending off for the old x-ray. Our major suspicion was that the "soft" shadow was cancer, but in view of his age, we postponed invasive tests hoping the prior film was still available. Fortunately, it was. As Jakowski had suspected, the dense nodule was clearly visible on the old x-ray—but so was the other spot as well, totally unchanged in size and character! Once again, my old adage had proven correct: "Brains are good, but old films are better."

The situation with Joe Felix was quite different. A productive business executive, he vigorously denied ever having been sick a day in his life. He watched his diet, exercised frequently, but drank and smoked almost to excess. He was about to retire. His wife encouraged him to have a thorough medical exam, and as part of it, a chest x-ray was taken. It was abnormal; a spot the size of a pea was noted near the top of the right lung. A TB skin test was also positive. But Felix was adamant that there was nothing wrong with him, and he resisted further investigation. His physician suggested watchful waiting for this tiny a spot, which was reasonable, but he also suggested a referral to us for consultation, which Felix accepted.

Felix was a striking man. Big, broad shouldered and muscular, he had an unusual face: the bony brow above his eyes was prominent with bushy eyebrows, his chin jutted forward, his hair hung down along the back of his neck. The adjective "leonine" was never more appropriate. I could ascertain nothing of importance in his present or past history or the remainder of his exam. He did, indeed, seem entirely healthy. And he denied ever having had a prior chest film.

I reviewed his x-rays. The tiny spot was real; it was visible on multiple views. It could have represented almost anything from the residua of an inflammatory condition to an aggressive tumor. In these days before CT scanning, tomograms were taken. In these specialized x-rays, "slices" of the lung were taken from back to front, but they didn't really help in this case. I could see the spot: its edge was a bit denser than elsewhere, which tended to reassure me that it was an inflammatory shadow, but that was still a speculative conclusion. Nevertheless, I leaned towards a benign explanation for the shadow.

I went back to the original chest x-ray and examined it even more carefully, following my "Look all over" principle. I noticed that on his left side, down low, three ribs revealed evidence of healed fractures, three in a row. Single fractured ribs are common, the trauma causing them sometimes so minor that they are not recognized by the individual. But when a number of ribs are cracked in a row, the common cause is an automobile accident or a more major injury.

I went back to Felix. It took some prodding, and it was actually his wife who remembered: two years previously Joe had been up on a ladder repairing their roof, and he had slipped and fallen. When his side kept bothering him, he had gone to his local hospital a few days later, and an x-ray had been taken. They had told him he had bruised some ribs.

Mrs. Felix left abruptly. She went directly to their hospital, obtained the x-ray, and brought it to us. The freshly fractured ribs were there, all right, but the right upper lung appeared to be absolutely clear. So this tiny spot had appeared within the last two years. Cancer suddenly became the likely diagnosis.

Surgery was performed; Joe's right upper lobe was removed, and indeed, the nodule was cancerous. Lung cancers of this size have the most favorable outcomes; in some studies more than half of the patients with them survive. Such was not the case with Joe Felix. Within a year evidence of the cancer having spread to his liver occurred, and he succumbed.

Joe's case succinctly demonstrates the benefit of examining old and new x-rays. But it also serves to underscore the point that the best option for lung cancer prevention is to stop smoking, or better still, never to start.

Hey, Wait a Minute

Harold Kunstler came in with a history of hemoptysis. A smoker, he said he had a chronic cough, sometimes accompanied with bloody expectoration, and had experienced such for about two years. He reported a few "chest colds" during the same period. He had not lost weight, and he did not look chronically ill. I could not hear breath sounds over his right lower lobe on physical examination, and his x-ray confirmed abnormality in the area. It showed a pancake-like shadow compressed medially up against the heart shadow, which I knew from prior experience suggested a collapse—a marked reduction in volume—of the right lower lobe. I could see no mass, but I knew the most common cause of such a change would be something such as a tumor growing within the bronchus to that lobe. Such a mass would then obstruct the airflow to the lobe and cause it to lose volume.

Bronchoscopy was performed by the surgeons using the rigid metal tube standard at that time. The bronchoscopist said he saw a tumorous swelling in the expected area, and he biopsied it. When we reviewed the case at a conference, the pathologist, who had studied the biopsied material, said, "Sorry, but you only got cartilage." Snickers were heard in the audience. The bronchial tubes are supported by rings of cartilage; sometimes, when biopsies are done, the abnormal structure is missed altogether, and the specimens only show normal bronchial tissues, such as cartilage. It was assumed such had happened, which explains the snickers.

"Now, wait a minute." The bronchoscopist spoke. "I saw a tumor mass. I have no doubt that I biopsied it. If all you see is cartilage, it must be part of a tumor." And so it was. We removed the offending lobe, and in the bronchus to it we found a marble-sized pearly nodule entirely made up of cartilage. Termed a chondroma, it is a rare, but well known, benign tumor of the airways.

I was visiting Kunstler at his bed while he was recovering when his wife, whom I had not met before, came in to see him. "I am so glad you removed that lung," she said, "that man has been coughing up blood ever since I've known him."

"Oh, are you just recently wed?" I asked.

"Oh, no," she replied, "next month will be our tenth anniversary." I questioned her further and learned that a decade earlier Kunstler had been seen with the same complaints at a major teaching hospital in a nearby city. I obtained a summary of his hospitalization from them. Unlike most summaries today, it was succinct. I can remember it clearly.

Complaint—hemoptysis

X-ray—Collapsed right lower lobe

Bronchoscopy—mass right lower lobe

Biopsy—cartilage only

Diagnosis—hemoptysis of unknown etiology

My smile was ironic. I could, in my head, hear the same snickers at the other hospital years ago. Unfortunately, their bronchoscopist had not said, "Hey, wait a minute." Fortunately, all that was lost was a decade; what was gained was a great case for a lesson in a bronchoscopist's confidence and perseverance.

First Week in July

I was sometimes asked to review pending medicolegal cases, ordinarily on the side of the defendant physicians. Following my review I would offer the attorney my opinion about the likelihood of success or failure in the case, coupled with advice as to settling or proceeding with it. I am proud to say my advice was usually taken; sometimes a case progressed to deposition and to trial.

I found many plaintiff lawyers quite reasonable in their conduct and in the cases they took; only a few fulfilled the stereotype of the predatory plaintiff attorney pushing unwarranted claims in hopes of a commercial settlement. One such case concerned an elderly Hispanic man, Jose Valentina, whose wife had died of lung cancer the prior summer at the University Hospital. The suit was filed against the community hospital, where she had been seen for many years for cardiac symptoms and findings. The complaint was that the lung cancer diagnosis had been missed at her hospital, so her physicians and the hospital were therefore guilty of negligence and malpractice.

I had access to the records and x-rays from both hospitals for review. At the community hospital her chronic heart failure, I thought, had been managed well. I also agreed with the hospital interpretation of her chest x-rays, right up to her last admission there, six months before her death. The x-rays showed evidence of the heart disease. They were otherwise normal, except for some prominence of the aorta, the major blood vessel that leaves the heart to begin the transport of blood to the rest of the body. Specifically, and most importantly, there was no sign whatsoever of a tumor.

Only a few months later, Mrs. Valentina had shown up at the University Hospital with a new set of symptoms. Her x-rays at that time were markedly different, revealing a large melon-sized mass of tissue in her right lung adjacent to, and probably spreading into, her mid line structures in the region of the aforementioned aorta. Studies confirmed an undifferentiated large cell lung cancer; given the normal x-ray only six months before, the giant size of the mass established it as a rapidly growing tumor. Not surprisingly, it was soon fatal.

I could not understand why the suit had been brought; I was even more surprised when it went to trial. I felt sorry for Mr. Valentina, the plaintiff, who sat forlornly next to his smartly dressed attorneys, understanding little of the proceedings. In cross examination his lawyers unsuccessfully attacked my credentials; they then presented me, one by one, with the names of the patient's University Hospital physicians and asked if I knew them and their excellent reputations, which I did—until the final name, one Dr. Laskowski. This was a new name for me, and I said so. In fact, I did not even remember seeing his name in the chart. They then proceeded to ask me why, if I was so certain this was a rapidly growing cancer, the University had thought it present for years? I was bewildered; I responded that not only did I not know, but that I doubted any of my colleagues had felt that way. I said there existed no evidence to support "present for years," and I was able to show the jury the difference in the final x-ray at the community hospital, and the first one at the University. To my pleasure, the jury decided for the defendants.

I, however, remained confused. Where, I wondered, did these aggressive attorneys get the idea that the tumor was of long standing, and therefore, had been missed at the first hospital? It could not have been because the shadow of the aorta was mistaken for a tumor; no one would have made that simple error. To attempt to satisfy my own curiosity, I decided to review the chart again. And then, a discovery: it was the death certificate. She had died at 3:00 a.m. on July 5th and the death certificate was signed by a Dr. Laskowski, obviously a brand new intern on call that night. He was called in to pronounce the patient deceased and to fill out and sign the certificate. Death certificates have a place to describe the immediate and basic causes of death, the contributory conditions, plus the duration of each. And there it was: "Pulmonary hemorrhage and insufficiency, duration hours; due to bronchogenic carcinoma, duration *years*" (italics mine).

A new intern, at night, not knowing anything about the specifics of a case, had relied on his basic knowledge, which was that lung cancer was ordinarily a relatively slowly growing neoplasm. The attorneys, when going through the records, combing through every action and word for a possible error, had grasped onto the word "years." Naturally, they had assumed it represented the combined wisdom of the staff at the University, rather than the hasty word choice of a harried new physician.

It used to be recommended that one do one's best not to be hospitalized in July, because that's when new interns and house officers come on board. To my knowledge, there is no evidence to demonstrate that mortality or complication rates are higher during this period. In our hospital, in fact, the attending physicians involve themselves even more directly in patient care at this time; nevertheless, the prejudice remains in some quarters. I doubt anyone ever had in mind the risk of a misleading death certificate. Even after this singular Valentina experience, I cannot say it has ever been, or should be, a serious concern.

Aunt Minnie, and the Sin of Pride

Benjamin Felson, a justly renowned radiologist from Cincinnati, wrote a marvelous little volume on chest x-ray interpretation. In the introduction he relates an anecdote:

A man says, "Look over there, there's Aunt Minnie."

He is questioned, "How do you know it's Aunt Minnie?"

To which the man responds, "Why, look at her—surely it's Aunt Minnie—who else could it be?"

201

Felson decried the overuse of this method for x-ray interpretation—the "Aunt Minnie approach." Today it is more elegantly termed "pattern recognition." I felt the same way about its overuse and, in fact, in my own approach to diagnosis and teaching, I used many of Felson's principles. I believe the combination of both clinical and x-ray findings is more helpful in diagnosis than simple pattern recognition, particularly since pattern recognition alone would never permit one to diagnose an entirely new condition. That said, however, there are some circumstances in which the appearance of a condition on an x-ray is so typical and unique that recognizing the metaphoric "Aunt Minnie" is the correct and most efficient approach.

Heinrich Gottlob is one such case in point. Gottlob owned a farm in one of the townships surrounding Ann Arbor. His ancestors were early German settlers in Washtenaw County, and Henny, as he was called, had maintained the family tradition of hard work on the farm. He had lost two fingers in an accident with some sort of farm machinery. This always made shaking his hand an unusual experience for me.

Working in the field one afternoon, Gottlob, a healthy and sturdy man, had suddenly and unexpectedly expectorated a handkerchief full of bright red blood. A veteran of World War II, he promptly came to the VA Hospital. A chest x-ray was taken; it showed advanced changes throughout the right half of the chest. Gottlob was immediately admitted to the hospital and placed in isolation on my tuberculosis ward.

When I came to the hospital the next morning, I was informed of Heinrich, and his x-ray was shown to me. I could not suppress a laugh. It wasn't that the film wasn't abnormal, because it was. But it did not represent active tuberculosis. It did not even represent lung disease. Gottlob's x-ray revealed multiple irregular shadows, which were very dense along the lateral chest wall where they presented as a thick, dense, white shadow. The appearance was absolutely typical of a unique pathologic state—that of calcified pleural plaque. The pleura consists of thin layers of lining on the surface of the lung and the inside of the rib cage. It permits the lung to glide easily along the chest wall; the two separate layers offer a potential space in which air, fluid, or blood, for example, can collect. Some such conditions can result in pleural plaque.

(Note, the thick lateral band is seen as such, because all the changes from front to back along the side of the chest are now seen on end.) Pleural plaque is absolutely paramount among the "Aunt Minnie's," especially when calcified. (The case described in "More Sinned Against" is an example of the tragic errors that can occur when the shadow is not properly diagnosed.)

Calcified pleural plaques of this type are usually the end result of remote infection or bleeding into the pleural space. I removed Gottlob from isolation and then examined him. I asked about prior illnesses and was able to confirm his story by review of his service records. It turned out that while in service, Gottlob had experienced an overwhelming infection of both belly and chest, in which pus had been present in both his peritoneal and pleural spaces. A firm cause had not been established, but the possibility of a number of specific infections, including tuberculosis, had not been excluded. In any case, the history was an adequate explanation for the pleural plaque. Gottlob's tuberculin skin test was positive, indicating prior infection, but not necessarily disease, due to the TB germ. And in fact, the CT scan, now available, showed no disease whatsoever in his lungs. If the prior illness had been tuberculous, this meant that Gottlob was at high risk for relapse. As a precaution, I prescribed isoniazid, the potent anti-tuberculosis drug, as prophylaxis against future relapse. Today we would call Heinrich's situation "latent tuberculosis" and treat it the same way.

But wait—we still had the hemoptysis, the blood spitting, to explain. The lining of Gottlob's upper respiratory tract—nose and throat—was unrevealing. We proceeded to bronchoscopy to examine the lining of all his airways. The procedure is ordinarily performed by one of the pulmonary fellows with a staff physician supervising, and so it was with Gottlob. Frankly, somewhat to my surprise, since many bronchoscopies for hemoptysis are normal, we saw a tiny, bright, cherry red mass protruding from one of the branch bronchi to the right lower lobe. It was another Aunt Minnie: the appearance was absolutely characteristic of a specific type of tumor of the airways called a bronchial adenoma. Any such impression, no matter how strong, should be confirmed by biopsy and tissue examination. But therein lay another problem. Adenomas are notorious bleeders when biopsied; we prodded it gently, and "washed" it with saline solution. Fortunately, it did not bleed, and even more fortunately, our pathologist was able to confirm from the washings that this was, indeed, a bronchial adenoma.

We next faced the problem of what to do. Most adenomas are "benign" in the sense that they only grow locally and do not spread elsewhere—but a small percentage of them do, and a patient who has one is always subject to recurrent bleeding, which can be massive. The recommended form of treatment is usually surgical removal of the tumor along with the lobe or segment of the lung in which it lies. However, for Gottlob, the calcified (presumably obliterated) pleural space would make such surgery horrendously difficult and possibly fatal.

I consulted with one of my colleagues at the Mayo Clinic who had much experience with a special technique for treatment and removal of these tumors through the bronchoscope. He agreed that Gottlob's was too small and too far down the airway for this procedure to potentially be successful. After much thought and discussion, it was agreed that we would reexamine the tumor via bronchoscopy every six months or so. We had been unable to see it on the CT scan, even knowing where it was, but decided to repeat the CT scan at intervals as well to observe any change. Heinrich was agreeable to this approach. He seemed a solid citizen, who would be reliable in reporting any bleeding or change in his condition.

Our cautious approach provided us with an additional unplanned educational benefit. Adenoma is not a common tumor, so for many years, almost a generation of pulmonary fellows in training had the opportunity to see for themselves the appearance of a typical confirmed adenoma! I was also pleased to reassure myself every six months that there was no change. Still another benefit to Gottlob's semi-annual examinations was that I became better acquainted with him and appreciated his stalwart personality. It might be stretching it to say we were friends, but he and I were more than just acquaintances.

Six years passed. Then one day when Gottlob reported for his now routine bronchoscopy, I, more or less subliminally, noticed a peculiar, somewhat foul odor in the bronchoscopy suite during the procedure. It did not fully register in my consciousness at the time; the adenoma was unchanged, and by the time we had completed the examination I had forgotten about it. The x-ray taken that day was also reported to have shown no change; for whatever reason, it was a week or so later before I reviewed it myself. This review was standard, somewhat compulsive behavior on my part, behavior that went back as far as my tuberculosis sanatorium days when I read all my own x-rays and became accustomed to doing so for all of my patients. It was also probably due to some arrogance on my part, since I believed I was more competent in chest x-ray interpretation than many radiologists. And the third reason was because of my special relationship with Gottlob and his special case. Superficially, the x-ray did appear as it had for years; but, as I continued to study it, I became convinced that there had been a subtle change. Some of the irregular calcifications at the right base seemed to have shifted ever so slightly in position towards the center of the chest. Minor changes in the position of the patient and the angle at which the film was taken could cause minor shifts in shadows. I put the film aside to review afresh a few days later; upon this second review, I convinced myself the shift and the changes were real.

The question was why? Some new pathology could be pushing or pulling the calcifications, but I saw no new shadows to account for such a shift. Before I proceeded further I felt I needed some confirmation of my apparent certainty; the radiologists at the VA disagreed with me, and once again my belief in my own competence had led me to have little respect for most of those at the University. The exception was Dr. Barry Gross, who specialized in chest disease, and whom I considered a superb diagnostician. Unfortunately, Gross had moved to Henry Ford Hospital in Detroit. I called to set up an appointment to see him and review the x-rays with him; he was out of town at a meeting. Then, it was one thing after another: the holidays came and went, I was busy on service followed by a scheduled vacation, we both had meetings. To bring the matter to a head, it was almost four months before we met in his office in Detroit. Oh yes, Barry said, I think you are right, I agree those calcifications have shifted. I was immensely gratified—but now I had to more seriously address the question of why. I decided to call Gottlob in for a CT scan.

Upon my return to Ann Arbor from Detroit I reviewed Gottlob's chart. A few weeks before that bronchoscopy, he had had a deep "chest cold." This had not been reported to me. When he arrived, Henny said he had not been feeling well all these months. He had experienced some chest pain on the right side, occasional fever, and a bad taste in his mouth. I now remembered that foul smell in the bronchoscopy suite. Stoic Gottlob had not returned to the hospital, because "I really wasn't that sick, doc," and besides, there was the farm to attend to.

With a sense of foreboding, I repeated the x-ray and the CT scan. A large grapefruit-sized shadow of fluid density now occupied a zone between calcifications at the right base. Despite the massive scarring, it now appeared that Gottlob's pleural space had never been completely obliterated. Following the apparent pulmonary infection months before, the residual space had once again been infected—or, forty years later, the prior pleural infection had relapsed—and another massive collection of pus—an empyema—had occupied the pleural space. Antibiotic therapy alone would be inadequate to treat this complication. Other questions now arose: what was the relationship between the adenoma and this new development? Had the adenoma obstructed or interfered with normal defense mechanisms in that lobe? Had pneumonia developed behind it, which led to the empyema? Bronchoscopy showed no change in the tumor. Major surgery would now be necessary to drain the pus, but could the adenoma be dealt with surgically at the same time? No—drainage of the pus required a difficult, extensive surgical procedure in which much of the chest wall, including ribs and pleura, had to be removed. As it was urgent to drain the pus first, this complex operation was performed. Attacking the lung at the same time in a contaminated operative field was considered too risky.

Gottlob tolerated the procedure well. He returned once more to the farm, and to future surveillance of the adenoma.

I was pleased that I had correctly recognized the subtle change in the calcification's shift, but my pride and my competitiveness had blinded me to thinking the situation through. My behavior had an aspect of what is called "search-satisfying bias"—a tendency to stop looking for additional explanations or diagnoses, once a seminal observation or diagnosis is made. I surely should have asked myself what could have moved those calcifications over. Had I coupled my observation with the chest cold and the smell in the bronchoscopy suite, I might have suspected the possibility of the empyema. And, as my colleague Milton Gross pointed out, a number of radioactive scans were available which could have located the accumulation of white blood cells present in the collection of pus. A less extensive procedure might then have been done.

Not for the first time, it was I who learned an important lesson. My sin of pride had otherwise marred what could have been a superb example of a sophisticated exercise in diagnosis and treatment. It demonstrates how theoretically irrelevant emotions can interfere with the practice of medicine, even when one has the best of intentions. Certainly a good lesson worth teaching!

Some other Aunt Minnies

John Brady was an alcoholic who entered our hospital with fever and left-sided chest pain. His physical exam showed multiple signs of his drinking problem and its damage to his liver; additional findings suggested the possibility of fluid in his left chest. His x-ray, however, was startling. Indeed, there were changes at the base of the left lung compatible with a fluid collection, but far outweighing that was a giant volleyball-sized space of some type at the base of the right lung. It had a thick irregular wall and a level line running across it, which represented an air-fluid interface. The medical term for this shadow is an "air fluid level." It implies that, whatever the cause, fluid is collecting and cannot be completely eliminated despite the apparent connection to the air in the outside world. The appearance on Brady's x-ray was remarkable and unique—none of us had ever seen anything exactly like it.

What could it be? Our first thought was a giant lung abscess. But if that were so, we would expect a lot of sputum expectoration, and Brady had none. Could it be an empyema—a collection of pus and air in the pleural space? If that were the case, Murphy should have been horrendously ill, which he was not. Could it be a giant excavated cancer of the lung? If so, it would have been growing for a long time, and Brady seemed too well for that. We were stumped.

207

I will not go through the diagnostic maze through which we stumbled; suffice it to say that, eventually, the shadow turned out to be Brady's stomach! "Turned out" is an apt phrase. The stomach, ordinarily a left-sided structure, had somehow twisted and repositioned itself so that it was located *above* Brady's liver. Specifically, it was now between the liver and the diaphragm, the muscle which separates the abdomen from the chest. Presumably it had found this bizarre location congenitally, although we could not be certain. Brady denied any symptoms that might relate to its change in position. We were fortunate that one of the procedures we had not attempted was a needle aspiration of the fluid. Had we done so, we might not have recognized the fluid as gastric juice, and tragedy might have occurred if some of the gastric contents had spilled into the abdominal—or pleural—cavity.

Oh, incidentally, the left-sided pleural effusion, the condition we had almost overlooked in our excitement about the shadow, turned out to be due to tuberculosis. Brady was treated, discharged, and then disappeared from follow-up, taking his unique anatomy with him.

Both before and after World War II, when tuberculosis was more common than it is today, mobile vans with fluoroscopic x-ray equipment would appear at schools and factories and elsewhere, offering to take mini films in an attempt to diagnose cases of tuberculosis early, even before symptoms had developed. The films were developed on long rolls, and read sometimes days or weeks after they were taken. "Lick TB; Get an X-ray" was a common slogan of the time. People did not need to remove their garments, and remained in street clothes while the films were taken. I remember an exhibit from a major urban health department shown at a national meeting in which a variety of remarkable items in the clothing, including firearms, were found. Some films, often without answers, were presented in a popular session at many meetings.

At one meeting of the Michigan Thoracic Society an x-ray with a bizarre undiagnosed finding was displayed. After many comments were made from the floor, I rose and not only said that the condition was a right-sided stomach, but also that the patient's name was John Brady, as indeed, it was. Talk about an Aunt Minnie!

###

Louis Grout was referred to us from a smaller nearby VA Hospital, bringing his x-rays with him. Dr. Robert Johnston, my fellow, saw him in clinic. The films showed a large, hazy, mass-like shadow in the lower medial portion of his right chest, adjacent to his heart. Multiple diagnostic procedures including bronchoscopy had been negative. Bob called me to the clinic, and we reviewed the x-rays together. On one, an oblique x-ray taken during a bronchogram, I could not identify the mass for certain. To me this was an Aunt Minnie; it suggested we were dealing with an intermittent (reducible) hernia of abdominal contents into the chest. The hazy character of the shadow suggested it was only omentum, the fatty apron that covers the abdominal organs. And the location implicated a specific potential track, termed the hiatus of Morgagni. A CT scan, which would have proved the herniated material to be of fatty density, would have been diagnostic, but CT scans were still far in the future. Instead, we took Mr. Grout to our procedure room where, with his consent, Bob performed an initial pneumoperitoneum, infusing air into the peritoneal cavity, just as I had done so often in my days in Talihina and for John Oriskany. We stood Mr. Grout up and took a chest x-ray. Sure enough, air entered the hernia space, thus establishing the diagnosis even before admission. You can bet the task of interpreting Mr. Grout's standard chest x-ray upon admission— which now contained free air in the abdomen—caused some consternation in the x-ray department, until we were able to explain the circumstances!

Many patients' x-rays have slightly different features in either structure or disease, which makes specific recognition of them fairly easy, particularly if the patients are seen and cared for over long periods of time. The ability to recognize individual x-rays is important for many reasons, not the least of which is the occasional misfiling error in which one patient's x-ray is placed in another patient's jacket. It was remarkable to me how often young physicians in training would fail to notice the various identifying differences. I would teach the importance of developing this skill, often concluding with the admonition that the x-ray features of one's long-term patients should become so familiar that one should be able to call the x-ray by the patient's name, as I did previously with John Brady.

To emphasize this point, I also had another favorite example. One of the faculty of our Dental school had studied Egyptian mummies by x-ray to evaluate the degree of tooth decay and other abnormalities. Some of these films were published, including a whole body x-ray of the mummy of one of the Pharaohs named Seti. I would show a facsimile of the picture of this mummy (in which the lungs had been removed and replaced by some foreign material) and ask not only for identification of the situation, but also for the name of the individual. Admittedly this was perhaps carrying the Aunt Minnie concept a bit too far!

###

One of my most popular teaching sessions held weekly involved demonstration of how to analyze a chest x-ray expertly. I would put up a chest x-ray on the view box and ask one of the residents, later the fellows, to analyze it. Although stressful for the participants, most found it valuable, as it tested not only their powers of observation, but also their methods of analysis and synthesis. The lessons learned when being expected to contribute their analysis under pressure tended to be more firmly fixed in their minds, than if they were merely observing.

Dr. Joel Seidman was a first-year house officer when he, himself, had a spontaneous pneumothorax. In this condition air from the lung, via one route or another, leaks into the pleural space, thereby collapsing the lung; fortunately, in Seidman's case it was only a partial collapse. I was involved in Seidman's care during this episode, which resolved spontaneously. Three years later Seidman was a pulmonary fellow, and in one of my teaching sessions I put up an x-ray of a left-sided pneumothorax; I called upon him to analyze it. He recognized the pneumothorax with no difficulty. I pushed him: "Do you see anything else?" This went on for a few iterations, as he recognized more subtle findings: there was air in the mediastinum (the tissues in the middle of the chest between the two lungs), and even in the pericardium, the tissue envelope that lines the exterior of the heart. But I still was not finished: "Surely you recognize something else?" Seidman did not. I then removed the label covering the patient's identifying information, and there was the name: Joel Seidman. I had shown Aunt Minnie her own film, and she had not recognized it. Joel, now a distinguished pulmonary physician here in Michigan, and I laugh about it to this day.

Lucille Garrison noted the recent onset of cough. She lived in northern rural Michigan, where a chest x-ray in a nearby town was obtained. It was remarkable. A grapefruit-sized mass sat at the top of each lung. The one on the right had an air-fluid level across it. A CT scan was taken which more clearly demonstrated the unusual abnormalities. The radiologist who interpreted the x-ray clearly had no idea of what was going on—his report mostly revealed his ability to fantasize.

Mrs. Garrison was referred to the University Hospital when I was on service. I recognized the abnormalities as Aunt Minnie's immediately. In the old TB days certain patients had received extrapulmonary plombages, procedures in which various materials, including Lucite balls and different waxes, were placed into the chest in an attempt to collapse upper lobe tuberculous disease. Lucille had had bilateral paraffin installations fifty years earlier; the one on the right had now broken through and established a connection to a bronchus, which had led to her cough and to the air fluid level. Her situation called for a relatively easy fix: removal of the plombages.

Mrs. Garrison's original surgery had also been performed at the University Hospital. She and I had very pleasant, rather nostalgic conversations about the physicians and surgeons we both knew from those days.

I faced a contrasting case at a Chest Conference a few years before I retired. One of my faculty colleagues, Dr. Paul Christensen, one of my former fellows, displayed a single x-ray and called on me to analyze it. I had done this to him many times, and mimicking me, he refused to give me any clinical information whatsoever. I felt my competitive juices rise to meet the challenge, hoping to apply the logical approach to chest x-ray interpretation that I had taught for so many years.

The x-ray was bizarre and remarkably asymmetrical. The entire left lung was shrunken and diffusely replaced by multiple dense lines of scarring, many circular, as if they surrounded small spaces. The diaphragm was elevated, and the heart shifted to the left. A number of conditions could result in this appearance, but they ordinarily caused changes in both lungs. What was remarkable here was that the right lung appeared entirely normal. One unilateral cause of the finding could have been prior extensive radiation therapy directed to the left side of the thorax. However, I had always taught that in the presence of asymmetry, one lung could be abnormal, or the other—or both. (My aphorism for teaching this principle was "Frame that Asymmetry" after William Blake's poem, "The Tyger.") I studied the normal side more carefully. I then noticed an irregularity of the fifth rib on that side, presenting what I termed the "Resh" sign—the Hebrew letter resh has a smooth sweep, as does the rib cage. When that sweep is interrupted, a common explanation is a former surgical procedure on that side. And yet, if this patient had had a biopsy, it would have been performed on the abnormal left side. Unless—

Lung transplantation had recently been described at a few other institutions, but Michigan had not yet begun such a program. Could a transplant be responsible for the right lung appearing normal? It would surely explain the findings, including the evidence of surgery on this "normal" side. I decided on that as my diagnosis. To my delight, I was correct! It goes to show that pattern recognition, the "Aunt Minnie," can carry you only so far. For something one has never seen before, only a logical, principled approach will do.

Ah, youth

Despite the hard and stressful work and the long hours, the days of being in training are often glorious for most house officers. Just out of medical school, basic medical knowledge is fresh in one's mind; one is up to date with current and new developments; one's skills seem to be at the height of what is required. In short, one seems to know it all! The idea of needing to consult with others seems unnecessary, except when encountering a strange specialty. In the days when internal medicine had not yet become highly sub-specialized as it is today, such was the common attitude. If one is an internist, even one in training, one would surely view other internists, referring to themselves as specialists in a particular area of internal medicine, to be superfluous. And yet...

At one time bronchoscopy, the procedure of directly examining the trachea and bronchial airways of the lung, was performed through a rigid metal tube. Unlike today, when pulmonary internists—"pulmonologists"—use a flexible tube in what is now an outpatient procedure, then, bronchoscopy was in the province of the thoracic or nose and throat surgeons. As young internists might not realize, the procedure was stressful and was not to be ordered lightly. It required prior approval by a chest physician should a medical house officer wish a patient to undergo the test. Some young trainees found this requirement a nuisance.

One such medical resident, a young man who later had a brilliant research career, approached me saying, "Look, my patient has hemoptysis (bloody expectoration). He obviously requires a bronchoscopy; please just approve it, so we can move on rapidly." I said I was sorry, but I really felt I ought to see and evaluate the patient for myself. He agreed, begrudgingly, knowing the bronchoscopy would otherwise not be done.

I had expected to find an older man, probably a smoker with lung cancer. To my surprise, this patient was in his thirties, rather young for a cancer diagnosis. He had been having intermittent expectoration streaked with blood, accompanied by chest pain and some shortness of breath for a few weeks. He had smoked a pack of cigarettes a day since his teens, not an inordinately heavy or lengthy schedule. His chest x-ray did reveal a large localized density towards the outer portion of his left lung with some associated fluid within the chest cavity. However, rather than the round shape commonly associated with a lung mass, this shadow was more triangular, wedge-shaped, the wide base laterally, up against the chest wall. It easily could have resulted from a growth within the bronchus leading to the area, and this is what the young house officer felt certain was responsible.

When I examined him, I found a healthy appearing young Puerto-Rican man in some minor distress from chest pain over the abnormal area, and some shortness of breath. The physical findings over the lungs were unimpressive, as was the remainder of his physical exam, except that I noticed a trace of edema—swelling due to some fluid accumulation—

at his left ankle. This was an unusual finding in a young man, which suggested, among other things, the possibility of an obstruction in the veins of his leg for which there was no ostensible cause. I chatted with him further, asking all kinds of questions about his medical and personal histories in an effort to find clues. He was an automobile mechanic; he had experienced no injuries, either at work or during this icy January winter. He had, however, been home visiting family in Puerto Rico over the holidays. He had flown both ways, cramped in the coach section of the aircraft in what was a very long flight in those pre-jet days. At that time we were just beginning to recognize the association of the inactivity of long trips with venous clotting in the legs. This condition can be complicated by pulmonary embolism—the migration of thrombi (clotted material)—from the legs to the lungs. Indeed, his story and the x-ray findings were strongly compatible with this possibility, which subsequent studies confirmed. The outcome, after administering the appropriate anticoagulant therapy—"blood thinning"—was positive.

The requested bronchoscopy was never performed. A somewhat abashed young resident had, I hoped, learned three lessons: first, about the benefit of careful diagnosis and not jumping to conclusions; second, about the need for greater humility; and third, about the benefit of seeking a consultation within various divisions of internal medicine.

Years later, at the start of another academic year, I was discussing cases with my team, when a new fresh-faced house officer entered the room and interrupted our talk by asking, "What lung tumor can cause bleeding for eleven years?" I responded that it would surely be an unusual situation, and that if he had such a patient, we would be glad to consult with him.

"No, no, no need for that; can you just answer my question?"

"Well," I said, "the bronchial adenoma bleeds, and can be very slow growing." Without a thank you, he turned to leave. As he left, I doubt he heard my parting request to see the patient.

Fortunately, his supervising attending physician felt the need for a consultation. The patient, a middle-aged workman named Sponberg, did, indeed, have a long history of recurrent cough with hemoptysis— expectoration of blood. The amount of blood in most of these episodes was minor. Eleven years previously, he had been hospitalized for it at a neighboring hospital, where his x-ray had revealed a round nodule, about ½ inch in size, in his right upper lobe. No diagnosis had been established. His most recent episode of bleeding in which he raised a bowlful of blood had frightened him and led to his readmission. Now, so many years later, his x-ray showed that the nodule had grown to baseball size. The house officer's assumption that it represented a very slow growing tumor was not unreasonable. However, on careful examination of the x-ray, I could see an irregular crescentic line above the "mass." The appearance suggested an Aunt Minnie. I ordered a special so-called decubitus view, to be taken with Sponberg lying on the x-ray table on his right side. What I had expected happened: the relationship between the mass and the crescentic line had changed. In the decubitus view, it was still "above" the mass, but if one held the x-ray upright, it appeared to be at the shadow's left side. In other words, the mass was moving freely within a space of some sort with a crescent of air above it no matter in which position the patient was placed!

This condition is known as an aspergilloma, more popularly referred to as a fungus ball. Empty spaces can occur in the lung for many reasons, most commonly as the result of prior infections or from destructive or developmental changes. A certain fungus, the aspergillus, finds this situation conducive to setting up housekeeping within the space, where it can gradually enlarge and result in a mass ("ball") of fungal material. The condition is important for two main reasons, both of which Sponberg exemplified: one, it can be misdiagnosed as a tumor, and two, it can cause bleeding which, at times, can be massive and life threatening. We were able to achieve a successful outcome for Sponberg by surgically removing the lobe and the fungal material in its space.

I thought the young house officer would be embarrassed by his apparent arrogance; I was wrong. He was only mildly abashed. "You know," he said, "although most people mean a benign or malignant growth when they use the word tumor—and I confess I did—the word actually just means a swelling." He smiled. "And so it was." He left our program after one year; I hoped that some day he would learn the lesson of humility.

The VA and Private Medicine

Harold Ingebritsen was in his thirties when he was referred to our VA hospital in the late 1950s with prolonged "fever of unknown origin." This state was, and is, not a rare complaint, one which still, in fact, poses problems in diagnosis. Multiple specific illnesses which cause it can be classified into three diagnostic categories: infections, tumors, and inflammatory disorders of the blood vessels or connective tissues. Having been briefly hospitalized in a nearby city where studies had been unrevealing, Harold was referred to us in Ann Arbor.

His illness included widespread infiltrates in the lungs, enlarged internal lymph nodes and involvement of the gastrointestinal tract. The specifics of the studies which led to the correct diagnosis are not relevant to my point here; suffice it to say that a systemic fungus infection was suspected, and then confirmed as histoplasmosis by the presence in his blood of antibody reactions to the organism, *Histoplasma capsulatum*. That this common soil fungus could cause widespread infection and disease through a wide swath of the midwestern United States had not been widely recognized until ten years earlier; establishing the diagnosis when we did required an unusual and sophisticated approach.

Ingebritsen was treated with amphotericin-B, the major anti-fungal agent available at the time. It is a toxic medication, and the house officers referred to it as "amphoterrible." Nevertheless, Harold tolerated it, responded nicely and was discharged well. We continued to see him in pulmonary clinic for a few years, but he was then lost to follow-up.

Thirty years later I saw Harold again, as a "new patient" in my clinic. I recognized the name, however, and upon questioning he confirmed it was he. A habitual smoker, he now had classic symptoms of chronic obstructive pulmonary disease. His physical examination confirmed my impression, but I also noted a large operative scar on the back of his chest. I asked him about it. "Oh," he said, "they thought I had a tumor and took out part of my lung, but it wasn't a tumor."

Even without obtaining the records from the other hospital, I suspected—nay, I knew—what had happened. Ingebritsen's treated histoplasmosis had left him with a clear space in his right upper lung, a space alternately termed a "thin-walled residual cavity" or a "bulla." The space was of no particular functional or anatomic significance, other than presenting an x-ray abnormality. However, a certain different fungus, the aspergillus, was known to take up residence in such spaces and cause a fungus ball, as I described in Ah, Youth. Aspergilli could grow in other similar spaces, and in the sixties the condition, at first a rarity, became generally better known.

An aside: at that time the Postgraduate Medicine department of our Medical School often sent professors on tours to teach at community hospitals. We were usually presented difficult cases as unknowns on these trips. During one trip in the sixties, I was shown a case of a fungus ball that had been removed under the suspicion it was a tumor at two separate hospitals!

Back to Inbgebritsen: his records confirmed my supposition. The loss of the lobe and the normal surrounding lung tissue had added to his respiratory difficulty. But, I wondered, why had Harold, who had received such excellent care at our hospital turned elsewhere for his care for the "fungus ball?" I asked him this question directly. "Oh, Doc," he said, "I had money then."

His attitude reflected a common one that organized medicine, unfortunately, often encouraged. That is, that private, fee-for-service care was superior to other forms of care, including that supplied by the VA. I am sure comparisons could be made in specific locations in which that was true, but general evidence to support this attitude was never available. In fact, recent studies have shown that for many conditions, VA care is, in general, superior to other forms. Nevertheless, the prejudice in favor of private medicine, prevalent in Ingebritsen's time, still persists in many quarters today.

My personal experience is, I think, relevant to this issue. After my internship at Mt. Sinai, a superb private hospital, I went to the VA in the Bronx, where I found the medical care competitive with that at Sinai. The patients were split between World War I veterans, often indigent, and recent veterans of World War II, mostly vigorous and employed young men. At that time, unlike today, the VA did not require a means test as a priority to be eligible for care. Many veterans had other options, but they came to the VA for one reason only: because they knew the care they would receive was excellent. And so it was. And so it was later in Ann Arbor, where the staff consisted entirely of University faculty. Although the resources available could not compete with those at a university hospital, the care was nevertheless comparable.

Potpourri

Parke Willis and his Very Dead Tree

The biggest, deadest elm tree was in Parke Willis's backyard, two houses down from ours on Martin Place in Ann Arbor. I firmly believe it was the first tree to bring Dutch Elm disease to the neighborhood. It stood there, massive and lifeless, for years and years, infecting all the elms for miles around. At least that was my perspective.

One day Parke, a physician colleague, finally decided to cut it down. Not by calling in some professionals, oh no. He wanted to do it himself. He had his sizeable chainsaw, his ladders, and his two sons there to help. He was up in that tree, sawing away, all day long. At times you couldn't see him because of the dust, which floated around and then settled on Parke, his sons, his yard, his neighbor's yard, his neighborhood. It was a summer evening, and Parke and his boys worked on until dark.

About 3:00 a.m. my phone rang. It was Parke. He had gotten up to pee, and noticed that he felt feverish and unwell. He asked if I would come see him. I grabbed my stethoscope and went over, thinking that I was about to diagnose a case of human Dutch Elm disease. I knew there wasn't any such thing, but there always had to be a first. And his illness just had to be related to all that dust. Parke was upstairs, in bed. His temp was 103. I examined him. Even through he did not complain of cough or shortness of breath, to my surprise, his lungs were absolutely clear, clear as a bell, not one abnormal sound or squeak.

219

I was mystified. The epidemiology was so strong. The illness absolutely had to be related to his sawing away at that tree. And yet his lungs were clear. What could be going on???

Here again was a case in which my principle was correct, but my deduction wrong. I had ignored the obvious symptom and fact. The secret lay in his getting up to pee. While sitting on that tree, straddling those rock-hard ancient elm branches all day long, he had traumatized his prostate gland and had developed prostatitis as well as a urinary tract infection.

So much for the first case of human Dutch Elm disease!

What Gets Rewarded?

Bob Winfield called for help. He had been a medical student and a resident with me; he now worked as the Director of the University of Michigan Health Service. He had seen a young woman, a graduate student, who had shown up complaining of fatigue, aches, pains, and other vague constitutional symptoms. Bob had taken a chest x-ray. It was abnormal, and he and the radiologist had suspected tuberculosis. However, her skin test was negative, as was the rest of his work-up. He was perplexed. As a favor to him, would I see her at the TB clinic for a consultation? Of course I would.

Other than the fact that she was thin and appeared nervous, I found her physical examination without abnormalities. Specifically, her lungs were clear, but her x-ray was surely not. She had multiple spots and patches in the right lung, considerable disease, out of proportion to her general appearance of relative well being. Her left lung was entirely normal. I felt strongly that the condition best fitting with her findings was one called sarcoidosis. I thought that despite the fact that sarcoidosis is typically bilateral and symmetrical affecting both lungs. I reassured her, called Bob, and gave him my opinion.

He referred her to the University Hospital, where they performed a bronchoscopy to biopsy her right lung. It confirmed the suspected diagnosis of sarcoidosis. The options were to treat her with steroids, or observe her for a time to see if the disease would resolve on its own. She opted for the latter, and with time, it did resolve on its own, as is common in sarcoidosis.

I present this case less for her story or my acumen but more to bring up issues related to compensation for services. At that time the physician's fee for the routine procedure of bronchoscopy was $300, and the University Hospital physicians so charged the patient. There were additional hospital charges for associated services while she was cared for at the hospital. As both Bob Winfield and I were employed by our agencies—he, the Health Service, and I, the Health Department—neither of us expected nor received additional recompense, even though we were the ones to make the diagnosis and steer the case in the right direction. Bob was grateful to me for my help, and I to him for the opportunity to see this interesting patient.

While I provided the consultation more as a favor to Bob, this situation still raises an important point related to our current complex compensation and reward system. Technical prowess and procedures— mandated by private and public health care insurance agencies, including Medicare, and approved by legislators who represent societal attitudes— are more highly valued than is the thinking that leads to them. I believe our health care remuneration system requires modification and reform.

Pembine

Pembine is a small town in Northern Wisconsin: due east of it is the Menominee River, which separates Wisconsin from the Upper Peninsula of Michigan. And, at one time, the Four Seasons Club was located on an island in the river. This rustic private club offered sporting activities all year round. John Towey, the chief physician at the Copper Country Sanatorium (that's Country, not County, which nevertheless is the name of the county) in the Upper Peninsula was a member. In the 1930s and '40s the tuberculosis physicians in Minnesota, Wisconsin and Michigan recognized that their practices differed considerably. A certain patient in Minnesota would be treated with pneumothorax, while a similar patient in Wisconsin could receive a phrenic crush and pneumoperitoneum whereas the Michigan patient would likely end up with a thoracoplasty.

Starting in 1944 they decided to meet each fall at the Four Seasons Club, to hold a "consecutive case conference" to compare and discuss their practices. For example, one year they might choose patients with unilateral cavitary tuberculosis in the upper lobe as the specific topic for discussion. Three hospitals (or more), one from each state, were then charged to present ten consecutive new admissions starting on a specific date to see what was done and compare the results. Their purpose in comparing their differing approaches was, hopefully, by their subsequent discussion, to achieve general improvement in patient care. In the days prior to randomized control studies, this approach was a major contribution to medical education and practice.

The style at the meetings was remarkable: no holds barred. Nasty and often profane critical remarks accompanied by lots of laughter contributed to the overall feeling of camaraderie. This excellent educational arrangement was widely copied, and the model was called a Pembine type conference. I first saw the name when I was in Oklahoma, and remember having no idea what "Pembine" meant.

Rooms were limited at the Four Seasons Club, and it was only after I had been in Michigan for a few years that I was invited. I then became a regular attendee and presenter, and eventually a Michigan Chairman for a few years in the sixties. I was not able to attend during the years I served in the Dean's office of the Medical School, but subsequently resumed my attendance. I was very proud to present historical case material at the 50th anniversary conference in 1994.

The meetings started on a Friday, with the final session on Sunday morning. Friday night was "fun night," when participants brought unusual cases in an attempt, often successfully, to discumbobulate their colleagues. One afternoon was free for canoeing or whatever—mostly golf, as there was a nine-hole course going clockwise around the island. Saturday night in the basement bar usually involved beer, music, cards, jokes and singing. It was always a great weekend.

The conference still meets, every year, at a different location; perhaps

I simply reveal myself to be a product of my generation when I say that today the conference has lost much of the flavor of the old TB days.

A few presentations were always on disorders other than TB, but were always presented in the consecutive case format with presentations from each state. For variation, common topics, such as "Cases I wish I had never seen" and "TB cases that turned out not to be TB," sometimes offered comic relief. The cases presented were often remarkable, and the discussions always stimulating and instructive.

One specific case was presented by my friend and colleague JR Johnson. Dick had trained at Michigan and, in fact, had held a position comparable to mine at the Ann Arbor VA before he left for the VA Hospital at 2500 Overlook Terrace in Madison, Wisconsin. We were, thus, naturally competitive until he passed away a few years ago. One year, JR presented a case of a man admitted with what was obviously extensive tuberculosis in an almost totally destroyed right lung; his left lung was clear. His tests proved he had TB, but in addition, as I recall it, the sputum Pap smear, was also positive for malignant cells. At that point we all reviewed the materials and evaluated the situation. We all agreed the x-ray showed only TB, and that probably the Pap test was a false positive, an uncommon, but well-known finding. Great discussion ensued about what to do with general agreement that the TB needed treatment; the question of cancer required further observation, but no immediate action.

Dick then displayed the continuing x-rays. Although the patient improved clinically, his x-ray changed minimally. As was common in those days, and with no visible evidence of cancer, the right lung was eventually removed. In addition to tuberculosis, we all thought the pathologist might find a small hidden cancer in the resected specimen, but none was found. After the surgery, when follow-up x-rays were taken, we noticed a spot in the *left* lung that represented the cancer! In retrospect we realized our attention to and focus on the right lung had interfered with our seeing the shadow in the left lung which, although hard to see, had clearly been there. Dick then told us that that was exactly what had happened during the man's actual care at the hospital. The end result was, of course, disastrous.

223

This rather sad and unfortunate conclusion to Dick's story was naturally met with a somber gravitas among his listeners. At which point, Ben Lawton, a surgeon from Wisconsin, dared a remark: "Now I know why they call it Overlook Terrace." His timing was impeccable, and the joke worked as intended to relieve the solemnity. It was just this sort of black humor that was typical of the Pembine tradition.

This story also exemplifies another important point: that of the need to maintain a sense of humor, even in the darkest of situations. It is a crucial character trait that has helped many a physician cope in a profession where life-threatening situations are faced on a daily basis.

Errors

Much information has reached the public in recent years about both the frequency and tragic results of physician errors. For individual physicians, the problem is sometimes compounded because neither the patient nor the physician learns of it, or the error is never discovered. That surely must be true for me; some known slips in judgment are described elsewhere in this volume. Here I wish to describe a few others with which I have been involved.

During my residency one of my diabetic patients required an unusually large dose of insulin. Insulin is usually given in specially-marked syringes; however, this particular patient's dose was so large that a large ordinary syringe was required. At the same time another one of my patients was receiving a large dose of a narcotic for an advanced form of a painful lymphoma. One day the two syringes lay side by side on a nursing tray; inadvertently, the nurse switched them, so that the diabetic received the narcotic and the lymphoma patient, the insulin. The error was promptly recognized when the lymphoma patient became faint and broke out into a cold hypoglycemic sweat. The diabetic fell fast asleep; time and some stimulants resulted in no lasting harm for him. I wish I could say the same for the lymphoma patient. But unfortunately, despite massive infusions of sugar, we were unable to rescue him. The insult to his already weakened constitution led to his death.

224

Today, with modern labeling, such an error would be unthinkable, or surely, excessively rare. An additional safeguard lies in the now common procedure that the nurse or any health care worker will ask the patient for his or her name and birth date before instituting any procedure or injection. Errors, or course, can involve anyone in our hard-pressed medical care system. The immensity of volume and detail required from these dedicated professionals is, I think, not adequately appreciated by the public. The emphasis in the media in recent years has been on the unfortunate frequency of 'medical' error. I regret them, and any single error, as much as anyone; but I often think that even more remarkable and worthy of note is their relative rarity, despite the enormous load each and every health care worker carries.

The error in Jack Fine's case was quite different. Fine had severe chronic obstructive pulmonary disease with a prominent asthmatic component. I had cared for him for many years. I could not prevent the progression of his illness, but I felt I had kept him as functional as possible. An acute exacerbation of his condition had required the use of high doses of steroids—cortisone derivatives—known to have a strong anti-inflammatory effect on his exacerbation. At a regular clinic visit when he was doing well, I changed his prescription by starting a "taper": reducing, or tapering off his intake of prednisone from 40 mgm a day to this same dosage *every other* day, and I so instructed him. A month later, at his next clinic visit, to my surprise Jack limped in with a cane. This was a major change for him. He told me he had developed serious pain in both hips. His lungs were about the same. I asked about his medicines, and he told me he was taking the prednisone four times a day. What?!?— *Why?* He showed me his bottle of pills, and there it was clearly typed on the label: *take four times a day.*

"But Jake," I said, "don't you remember that I told you clearly it was to be every other day?"

"Yes," he said, "but when the bottle came labeled that way, I thought you must have changed your mind."

I was appalled, and frightened. Like many physicians, I still used

225

Latin abbreviations in my prescriptions. "Q O D"—"quod alta diem" stands for every other day; but "Q I D"—"quod intra diem"—stands for four times a day. Had I erred in writing my prescription? Or had my handwriting, unarguably poor, been so bad that it had been misinterpreted by the pharmacist? I rushed over to the pharmacy, where the prescriptions remained on file. I found it. There, clear as it could be, was my "O," which could not be read as anything other than that. I breathed a sigh of relief. It was now the pharmacist's turn to be appalled by the error. To Jake, of course, it made no difference who was responsible for the mistake; both of his hips eventually had to be replaced surgically. The outcome was distressing, but thankfully, not fatal.

My involvement as a consultant in medico-legal cases, as mentioned previously (with Mr. Valentina in "First week of July"), has offered me an opportunity to participate in a battleground at the center of which is medical error. I do not believe the current tort system is a fair, nor effective, method of dealing with medical malpractice; nevertheless, I was always willing to review cases for attorneys and advise them about the likelihood of the outcome based on the medical aspects of the case. I would then, if asked, accept certain cases representing the defendant physician, when I believed that neither negligence, nor malpractice, was involved. I was pleased that most of these were settled at the deposition level, rarely going to actual trial. Later, attorneys who had thus become familiar with me would ask me to intervene on the plaintiff's side. I accepted some of these cases, as it afforded me the opportunity to create awareness of errors that might be corrected or prevented in the future. I also could help achieve appropriate compensation for injured parties.

In one such case, the patient, a woman in her late eighties, was resident in a nursing home. She became acutely ill with heart failure. She was transferred to the hospital where her primary physician managed her care superbly. She was then returned to the nursing home. An extensive summary of her hospitalization was dictated.

When I was in training, I was taught that a summary of every hospitalization was necessary, both for the record and for transmission of information to other physicians. At that time we wrote short, succinct summaries. An extreme example would be: "Mr. Jones was admitted with x, which was confirmed by y tests. He received treatment with z and was discharged." Anyone requiring additional information would have to check the chart itself. More recently, however, the summary of the hospitalization has become a long narrative recording of everything in the chart, going on for many pages, much too long for the dictating physician to edit and correct. For this reason, errors could occur, as happened to this patient.

In this elderly woman's case, one of her discharge medications was a potassium supplement, microK 10 meq (milliequivalents per liter) twice a day, to replace the potassium lost due to the use of diuretic agents helping to rid the body of excess fluid. In her summary, however, the order was typed as *micronase* instead of microK. Micronase is an anti-diabetic drug. The staff at the nursing home knew its dosage was measured in mgm, not meq, the measurement for microK. So the staff changed the transfer order to read micronase 10 mgm. Despite a repeat retransfer history that indicated the patient had *no history* of diabetes, the doctor ordered and the patient received the anti-diabetic medication. This resulted in hypoglycemia and, before the error could be corrected, the woman's death.

Reviewing the records, I was disturbed at the failure of the summary to have been reviewed and corrected. I assumed the dictated word micro *k* had been heard and transcribed as micro *nase*. This appalling error was compounded by the fact that the medication was administered despite the patient's lack of history of diabetes. This all too common transcription error could easily be corrected by reviewing the summary carefully.

I am pleased to say that at least my intervention and interpretation led to a satisfactory settlement in the case. I know that the physicians and the nursing home staff involved in this case were more careful subsequently. Perhaps recounting the story here will help create more general awareness of the problem.

Benjy Gordon

From 1966 to 1970 I, and my entire family, went every summer to Camp Walden, in Northern Michigan. We were there the first year for two weeks, and the last four years for four full weeks. I was camp physician. I had heard about the opportunity from one of my pulmonary fellows, as the co-owner of the camp, Neal Schechter, was a distant cousin of his.

My responsibility was to be the doctor on the grounds and to run two sick calls per day, one in the morning and one in the evening. A nurse actually took care of most of the minor problems during the days. Serious cases were to be taken to the emergency room and hospital in nearby Cheboygan, so there was often little for me to worry about. I did set things up for the appropriate practice of medicine in what I considered a more satisfactory manner than I had originally found. For example, a major complaint in the summer at any camp is sore throat. Many are not serious, but if the *Streptococcus* is involved (strep throat), hazardous consequences might follow if the infection is left untreated. It is generally accepted that the clinical differentiation of viral from strep throat is not reliable, so the options a doctor has are to treat everybody with penicillin, to rely on clinical judgment anyway, or to check all cases with a test for strep. In those days the strep test involved a throat swab, the specimen mailed to the state lab for culture of the germ. A positive test diagnosed strep throat with almost absolute certainty, and a negative test similarly ruled it out. After my first summer I made arrangements with the state lab so that I, and all other camp doctors, could appropriately culture for strep throat and eliminate the guesswork from sore throat diagnoses.

One summer we had a minor epidemic of delayed chicken pox at camp. Benjy Gordon, a cute ten-year-old, turned up one evening complaining of sore throat. He had a few pox-like sores on his skin, and in his throat I saw a big typical pox lesion on one tonsil! The rest of his throat was not red, but I cultured it anyway. I gave him some topical medicines to soothe the throat pain. A few days later the culture report came back negative for strep; however, Benjy's throat was not improving and still quite sore. And, a few days after that, Benjy's parents appeared on the scene.

228

The Gordons were wealthy Detroit-area merchants and major supporters of Camp Walden; Benjy was the fifth Gordon to have attended the camp. His parents wanted to know: Why hadn't I given Benjy penicillin? I reviewed the situation with them, explaining that I was certain he did not have strep throat. Well, they had talked with their family doctor at home, and he had said Benjy should get penicillin. They insisted I give it to him.

It was a delicate situation, which raised a bunch of issues. First was the question of patient autonomy: does a patient or family have the right to insist upon a treatment the physician thinks inappropriate? What if the treatment requested, even if it will not be helpful, has only a small likelihood of being harmful? And then there are the financial considerations. In private practice, failure to cooperate with a patient's desires may lose you the patient. In this specific situation, I had no doubt a physician could easily be found to give the requested treatment. I, of course, faced no problem in losing the patient from my "practice;" however, being so discontented, these major financial contributors to Camp Walden might decide to take their "business" elsewhere. That my future employment at the camp might be affected was a minor issue compared to the impact on the camp itself. How was I, in microcosm, to deal with these broader issues?

I went to Neal Schechter, the camp director, since he might well be the one most affected by my decision. I explained the situation. I told him I was unwilling to give the penicillin and why, but that I wished him to know about the situation in advance. I do not know how I would have reacted had he requested that I give the penicillin anyway. Fortunately he did not. He simply told me to do what I thought was right.

I returned to the family, and once again, explained my position of why I was unwilling to give the penicillin. They did not seem terribly upset—I think they were expecting such an answer. They took Benjy out of camp, took him to a doctor in town and, as I had expected, he got his penicillin. A few days later Benjy was better. Of course, they assumed his improvement was from the shot. I expected it was from the natural course of the illness.

This situation illustrates a broader issue in medical practice as it relates to patient autonomy and the patient expectations that each doctor/patient encounter end with a prescription for a pill or a quick-fix injection. It was clear to me that maintaining my ethical standards was more important than appeasing any patient (who, in this case, were Benjy's parents) with an inappropriate request. Patient autonomy would not, and did not, trump my standards. And the Hippocratic principle of "First, Do No Harm" surely influenced my refusal to prescribe the unwarranted penicillin. I had gone to camp for a month of fun and relaxation with my family. Little did I expect that I would encounter a test of my moral integrity. While in the larger scheme of things, this was a minor incident, it, nonetheless, helped to confirm my own ethical standards in the practice of medicine.

Fun and Games

A common method for teaching pulmonary medicine through pulmonary radiology is to show a student an x-ray, and ask him or her to analyze it. The student can then ask questions about the patient, reevaluating the x-ray after each new piece of information, until a final diagnosis can be reached. Anyone subjected to this method, especially if it should occur during a group training session, is anxious under pressure and tries to be as thorough and careful as possible during the evaluation.

The abnormality on one such x-ray I often used was easy to see: it was a relatively thin walled cavity in the left upper lobe. Everyone would think of cocci (a fungal infection which causes this type of shadow); and if they looked carefully at the film they would notice the hospital identification marker in one corner at the top: Veterans Administration Hospital, Phoenix, Arizona—and that would clinch their diagnosis, as cocci is endemic there. In this case, the facts were that the patient had become ill with symptoms of a pulmonary infection in Missouri on the way from Michigan to Arizona to look for work. My teaching point—that it was unwise to jump to a diagnosis before having all the facts—was made. Upon arrival he had checked into the Phoenix VA where they, too, had diagnosed cocci.

The man's subsequent course had had an interesting component as well. Initially misdiagnosed, the infection had progressed to what appeared to be considerable destruction of the lobe. He returned to Michigan; after treatment he was left with a residual hole in the lung which we resected. At a conference immediately thereafter, we were told that the pathologist had diagnosed bronchiectasis. This condition is usually more generalized and involves the lower lobes. I disputed the diagnosis, suggesting that the infected cavity had been relined with normal bronchial lining, as sometimes occurs, and thus the structure resembled a bronchus—a diagnosis which was met with derision by several others present. When I reviewed the material myself, I realized the man had a congenital lesion, a so-called bronchogenic cyst, which had become infected and had inflated. Fortunately, the pathologist, when given adequate clinical information, also reviewed the slides and had come to the same conclusion. No matter; the original teaching point remained that one shouldn't jump to conclusions without all the facts.

For residents in training one stressful challenge is being asked to analyze a chest x-ray that is ostensibly normal. I used one such in another fun and games example, one which I had myself diagnosed correctly. I had searched all over: not only the heart and lungs, but also the shoulders, neck, abdomen, looking at every millimeter of the film, and everything looked normal. And, finally, I saw it. Radiology technicians were trained to affix a metallic "L," representing the left side of the body, onto the x-ray cassette to properly identify that side, since with some views, especially obliques, it could be difficult for some to be certain which side was which. But in this case, the "L" appeared to be on the patient's right side. The technician had not erred in the placement; the patient had situs inversus, a complete right to left malpositioning of otherwise entirely normal organs. I was able to make the diagnosis only by recognizing the apparent misplacing of the "L." So, the patient and his organs were normal, but the x-ray wasn't!

231

Talking about Cases

I naively thought it was probably specific for doctors, perhaps even only chest physicians, to talk to each other about their cases when they got together. One morning, at breakfast in a restaurant while my car was serviced, three men at an adjacent table were talking. They were electricians, apparently involved in major building construction. And what were they talking about? Obviously, cases—this experience, that experience, that problem, how unusual, what happened unexpectedly, what that person outrageously wanted—diagnostic and therapeutic problems. Change the content, and it could have been me speaking with my colleagues!

You never know where talking about cases will take you. Jerry Baum and I did it, and found we each had had a couple of patients in whom benign nodules in the lung due to the fungus which causes histoplasmosis had unexpectedly grown and simulated a tumor. That chat led to a joint publication of an article in the *American Review of Tuberculosis*.

When my wife and I were in London on sabbatical in 1981, her cousins came to visit. We walked in Hyde Park, near our flat on Westsbourne Terrace. An attractive older woman was walking her dogs nearby. "That's Ava Gardner," I said, to their uniform disagreement.

Challenged, I went up to her: "Miss Gardner?"

Here came the response, in a deep resonant tone: "Yes?"

My wife said when she heard that voice, she knew immediately I was right. Ava Gardner was very pleasant, and as a reward I had my picture taken with her.

Later that week I presented a lecture on CAT scanning in pulmonary disease at one of the major teaching hospitals in London. It was well received, and afterwards the Chief of the pulmonary section and I went to his office. We had sherry and talked. I was not surprised at all when he said, "Let me show you a case." The series of x-rays were actually quite interesting; the diagnosis was not firmly established, but probably was an unusual infection in a man who had been all over the world, in many strange and exotic places. Then on a label in the corner of one of the films, I noticed the patient's name: Stewart Granger.

"Stewart Granger?" I said—"is that *the* Stewart Granger?" (He was an actor, perhaps best known for his role in "The Prisoner of Zenda" opposite Deborah Kerr and James Mason.)

"Oh, yes," said my host, "he's a patient of mine."

"Well," I said competitively, "last week in Hyde Park I chatted with Ava Gardner."

"Oh," he responded, "she's also a patient of mine." (!)

And with that, he swiftly knocked me off my hubris. It was yet another reminder that one is better off letting humility, rather than conceit, guide one's actions.

At Journey's End

A Conflict of Roles

I doubt there is a doctor alive who has not been approached—at a party or some non-medical venue—by a friend or acquaintance with a request for advice. "Hey Bob, can I get your opinion on this?" "So I've had this pain...," or "I just read this article about my condition..." Most doctors surely handle this mild intrusion well, perhaps listening and commenting, if the issue is minor, or offering the name of a colleague for a referral, or perhaps even suggesting an office visit. A common conclusion to these encounters is a jocular, "You'll have my bill in the morning." Sometimes recipients realize the slight impropriety in their request; sometimes they don't.

To play the role of doctor for one's own family or among his friends is fraught with emotional complications which may impact judgment. Most physicians, properly, attempt to avoid that role—but not always with success.

Well into my career in Ann Arbor, a friend whom I'll call Janet Warner became ill. I knew her well—we were colleagues of long-standing and had been co-authors of a major publication. I knew that the alcohol she consumed—more than was moderate—had damaged her liver, but I was surprised to learn that she was hospitalized with obstruction to her stomach from a long-standing peptic ulcer. A standard surgical procedure became necessary and was performed.

Unfortunately, after a few post operative days, she developed a high fever, strongly suggestive of infection. The location of it was not apparent despite studies; she was treated with antibiotics without success. I had been visiting her regularly as a friend and was aware of the situation. Eventually her physicians felt strongly that she must have a hidden abscess somewhere: if they could locate it, it could be drained, which would be the proper treatment.

A new procedure, a radioactive gallium scan, in which the radioactive material localizes to areas where there are collections of inflammatory cells, such as in an abscess, had recently become available. The staff proposed the test, which required Janet's consent, but she refused. I was in no way involved in her care, yet her physicians whom I knew, and who realized we were friends, encouraged me to speak with her about it. I did. Why not have the procedure, I asked her. "Bob," she said, "if they do that radioactive test, it will kill me." I replied that the test was remarkably free of complications, and that a fatal outcome would be unheard of. I added my encouragement to that of her physicians. Finally, after a few more days of debilitating and drenching fever, she reluctantly consented. The material was injected—she promptly had a stroke, stopped breathing, and could not be resuscitated.

The autopsy found the abscess, near and in the tail of her pancreas. The cause of death was listed as a stroke. That may have been the mechanism, but I believe the real cause was the fear and anxiety which led her to will herself to death.

I was not part of her health care team; the surgeons felt strongly, correctly, that the gallium scan was important. I knew many of them, and when they realized I was her friend, they asked me to help convince her. The surgeons took advantage of our friendship, and I clearly overstepped the bounds in advising her. Obviously, the outcome was not "my fault"—I was not responsible for her death. Nevertheless, I was upset for my having confused the roles of friend and physician. I think I felt even worse, because I believed I had apparently not learned a very important lesson as well as I thought, that of "Listen to the Patient." Do you remember Mr. Rosenberg from way back in my internship? He was the man who also insisted he would not live if given insulin. Since that experience I held on to the "Listen to the Patient" dictum and even taught it in my classes. Yet here, with my friend, I did not apply that principle, nor did I associate the Rosenberg experience with my friend's own insistence, despite her using almost exactly the same words.

Medicine is a hard master. Hippocrates said it, millennia ago: Life is short, the Art is long, opportunity fleeting, experience misleading, judgment difficult. His wisdom was surely correct, particularly when judgment is clouded by emotion or bias. But then he added, "The physician must not only be prepared to do what is right himself, but also to make the patient, the attendants, and externals cooperate." And this is where I might disagree with my sage mentor Hippocrates. Sometimes, "to do what is right" is not to "make the patient" cooperate, but instead, to listen to a patient's own instincts.

The Patient's Right

My career as a pulmonary physician began as a tuberculosis specialist. The fascinating varieties of tuberculous infection could make dealing with this one disease satisfying for a lifetime. I expected a fulfilling career as a sanatorium director. Isoniazid changed the world and that expectation. The broader field of pulmonary disease proved to be an exciting and productive specialty for me. During my lifetime it evolved, and in the last years of my practice, I was heavily involved in critical care medicine and primarily dealt with acute life-threatening disorders in the intensive care unit. A far cry from the years of the long hospitalizations of tuberculous patients! Critical care medicine exposed me to a very different set of challenges, issues, and patients. One such patient, Jim Walters, exemplifies this.

As I entered my consultation room, I first saw Jim hunched over in a chair, head down, oxygen tubing in his nose, staring at the floor. His whole being epitomized dejection. During the interview it was hard for me to overcome my initial impression of him as a very depressed man. Jim was only in his late forties, but he had had progressive breathing difficulty for about five years. He had been cared for by a very competent chest physician in the private sector. A two- to three-pack a day cigarette smoker since he was a boy, the diagnosis was advanced lung disease, a mixture of chronic bronchitis and emphysema. Two years before, during an episode of pneumonia and an extreme exacerbation of his illness, he had been placed on a respirator; it was with great difficulty over many weeks that he could be weaned from the respirator. Despite further treatment with multiple medications, oxygen, and sophisticated physical therapy, his condition had inexorably progressed.

Walters and his wife were unusually knowledgeable about his situation and its treatment. Our conversation was pleasant and prolonged. I did not ask specifically why he had come to our hospital. It was common for veterans who had adequate health insurance, or who could afford private care, to seek it initially from a physician in private practice. For those in the latter class, however, the inability to work often led to gradual depletion of the family savings. They would then turn to the Veterans Administration for help. Walters was self-employed, and I assumed this was his situation.

As expected, my examination of Walters's lungs showed minimal movement of air in and out of his lungs, accompanied by abnormal sounds indicating obstruction to air flow with exhalation. These findings were typical for his condition. To my surprise I found that Jim's legs were massively swollen with excess fluid, right up to his knees. Walters said this was a recent development. This finding confirmed the seriousness of his condition. The lungs are placed strategically and functionally—though not anatomically—between the right and left sides of the heart. His advanced lung disease had led to increased pressures in the blood vessels of his lungs, and the strain had led to failure of the right side of his heart. This condition, termed cor pulmonale—heart disease due to lung disease—is often the serious end stage of that illness. One can predict with some confidence that death will occur within the next year or so.

When I commented on this finding, it turned out that Walters and his wife were both aware of how dire his situation was. We discussed his treatment; I told them I would prescribe some modifications of his medical regimen, and that there were a few new agents available we could try. I did not hold out unreasonable hope. They seemed content and agreed to work with us on his revised program.

On his next visit, a month or so later, Walters appeared more cheerful. His leg swelling had diminished. In response to one of my typical questions, they agreed he was "surely no worse," a construction I much preferred over suggesting to patients or encouraging them to say that they were "better." During this visit we talked about what would happen should he become acutely ill again. I explained that, with the degree of lung and heart damage he had, if his condition should deteriorate and he were put on a respirator, it would be very unlikely that he would be able to come off it and breathe again on his own. We discussed the possibility of making the decision now as to whether or not he wished to be placed on a ventilator, should that dire situation occur. I assured them I would, no matter what, remain fully involved in his care. I suggested they think about the issue and discuss it with whomever they wished—family, friends, counselors—before making a decision.

At his next visit Jim and his wife both clearly seemed more relaxed and, if not cheerful, more content. Walters signed a "DNR"—do not resuscitate—note in his chart. The note explicitly stated that, in the event of respiratory failure, intubation (a breathing tube) and mechanical ventilation were not to be used.

During the next year and a half I noticed little change in his status. Although "surely no better," his condition seemed to have stabilized. I was, therefore, surprised and indeed shocked to come into the hospital one summer morning to find Jim Walters in the intensive care unit on a respirator! He had been brought in by ambulance the night before, in extremis, and according to those who had seen him—and despite his prior decision—he and his wife had accepted the recommendation that he be intubated. It appeared that another pulmonary infection had pushed him over the brink with both lung and heart failure.

It is difficult for patients to communicate while on a respirator. Speech is impossible. For those who are alert, a pencil and pad permit the recording of their wants and comments. After a few days, with his wife at his side, I—gently, I hoped—broached the question of his decision to accept the respirator despite our prior discussions. Jim scrawled, "I have change [sic] my mind about this." His wife told me that the horror of the breathlessness had provoked extreme anxiety, and that he had grasped at the offered straw of the ventilator.

A week went by. Then two weeks more. Tests we label "weaning parameters" showed, as expected, that it was unlikely he would ever be able to be removed from the ventilator. We began considering the options. One was to perform a tracheotomy; the breathing tube would then enter his lungs from the neck, rather than from the nose or throat, which would make overall management easier. We would then transfer him to a facility for long-term chronic respiratory care. This was precisely the situation and life that both Jim and his wife had wished to avoid. Another option would be to optimize his condition as much as possible, and then remove the tube, giving him one more try at living without it. In this case the understanding would be that, should the trial fail, the tube would not be replaced and that Jim would die.

One morning, Jim and his wife asked me to remain after rounds. I did. They had talked about it; they wished to have the tube removed to see if Jim could survive without it. Faced with the reality of his situation in the emergency room, they were not sorry he had been put on the respirator. But now, faced with the reality of the future, once again their minds had changed. I agreed. Then Mrs. Walters said, "Dr. Green, we came to you as a last resort. We had been told Jim would die soon. But under your care he has had more than another year of life, and we are grateful. Now he is ready to go."

We maximized his status as best we could. As feared, but not unexpected, his attempt off the respirator failed. Jim died peacefully.

I learned a lot from the Walters. I photographed the sheet on which Jim had written, "I have change my mind about this" and made a slide of it, which I have often used in teaching. End of life issues remain serious, complicated and problematic. It behooves us all to remember that changing emotional situations may affect prior apparently rational decisions. The right to change one's mind, and then to change it back again, remains an inviolable patient right.

Epilogue

I have already described my journey from tuberculosis sanatorium director to critical care intensivist. During my sanatorium days I experienced deep satisfaction in living with my patients for months and years, getting to know many of them as individuals, not just as persons with disease. Reflecting on those years, and my entire career, I realize that for me, a major reward has always been the opportunity to form relationships with people like Betty Sue and Charlie Vandenbosch and Heinrich Gottlob and Elzie and the Walters, and so many others. Their personhood is inextricably linked to their illnesses, and the pleasure I experienced in helping them helped fulfill my own spirit.

I also had the privilege to be practicing medicine in an era of immense scientific discovery, innovation, and progress. The latter half of the twentieth century was ripe with many scientific studies—prospective multi-center randomized trials, of which tuberculosis chemotherapy was the prototype—which permitted us to be confident of the scientific validity of our therapies. Research from the bench was transmitted to the bedside. Our armamentarium was immense: antibiotics, vaccines, steroids, anti-inflammatory agents, anti cancer drugs, all became available in this era. We eliminated smallpox and came close to doing so for polio. We controlled many infectious diseases, including those most dangerous to children. We began to understand immunology, enzyme and protein function, cellular and molecular metabolism. New imaging techniques developed explosively. New specialties, such as geriatrics, clinical genetics, rehabilitation medicine, oncology, infectious disease, invasive radiology and cardiology, all began. Advances in anesthesia and surgery, not the least of which was organ transplantation, enhanced our ability to save and extend life.

I witnessed the changing structure of the profession as well, as this era of scientific progress was accompanied by social progress. The growth of employer-based and private health insurance programs, plus Medicare and Medicaid, assured that the majority of individuals could have access to excellent care, independent of their income. Many more options were available for physicians in terms of choice of career. One could still practice solo general medicine, the standard mode pre-war, but now a physician could also practice as a specialist, in a group, in academia, in industry, in research. My preference and choice to work as a physician with the Veterans Administration and the University was greatly influenced by my early training in the VA, and particularly by my years at the Indian Bureau Medical Center in Oklahoma. I felt privileged to provide high quality medical care to these less fortunate people who had fewer options for addressing their medical needs in the era of the pre-insurance private health care system. I was happy to be employed and salaried, and unconcerned with financial pressures; it was clear to me that I did not need the incentive of extra fees for my service to deliver excellent care. And thus, I continued in that mode for my entire career. I believe that personal financial considerations should have no place in the practice of medicine. I would challenge anyone who would claim that only-fee-for-service medicine delivers the highest quality of health care.

I retired from the University and the VA in 1995, although I maintained my connection with the Health Department for tuberculosis work for another decade. Towards the end of the century, satisfaction with practice declined for some medical practitioners, as they found bureaucratic requirements and the time-related pressures burdensome, even onerous. Regretfully, it seemed to me that the golden age of medicine had passed. It would no longer be as exciting and fulfilling for physicians in the twenty-first century.

Such a thought was quite naïve. Progress in cellular and molecular research, especially in the study of the human genome, continues to promise amazing opportunities for further advances in patient care and in the prevention and treatment of disease. I will miss being involved. I would be perfectly happy to begin the journey all over again!

242

My Promise

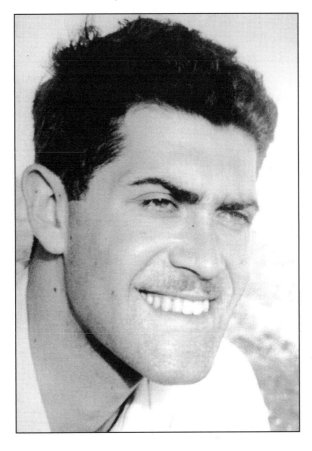

I took a position as ship's physician on the Panama Line for my two-week vacation during my year in Pathology. On the cruise down I cared for an elderly French Canadian woman whose diabetes was poorly controlled. She was grateful, and during the four days we spent in Panama and the Canal Zone she introduced me to her son and his family, who graciously hosted me. One day we went on a picnic out in the Panamanian jungle. They took my picture there. Shortly thereafter I met Lila, who became my wife; she loved the picture, and with a laugh said that if I ever wrote a book, it should appear on the back cover. I promised it would. It would be a bit misleading to do so now, so many years later, but my publishers kindly reproduce it here. Lila, I kept my promise!

Index